Practical Procedures in Anaesthesia and Critical Care

Practical Procedures in Anaesthesia and Critical Care

Dr Guy Jackson
Consultant Anaesthetist,
Royal Berkshire Hospital,
Reading, UK

Dr Neil Soni
Consultant Anaesthetist and Intensivist,
Chelsea and Westminster Hospital,
London, UK

Dr Christopher Whiten
Consultant Anaesthetist,
Charing Cross Hospital,
London, UK

Illustrations by
Jesse Brown

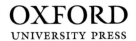
OXFORD
UNIVERSITY PRESS

OXFORD

UNIVERSITY PRESS

Great Clarendon Street, Oxford OX2 6DP

Oxford University Press is a department of the University of Oxford.
It furthers the University's objective of excellence in research, scholarship,
and education by publishing worldwide in

Oxford New York

Auckland Cape Town Dar es Salaam Hong Kong Karachi
Kuala Lumpur Madrid Melbourne Mexico City Nairobi
New Delhi Shanghai Taipei Toronto

With offices in

Argentina Austria Brazil Chile Czech Republic France Greece
Guatemala Hungary Italy Japan Poland Portugal Singapore
South Korea Switzerland Thailand Turkey Ukraine Vietnam

Oxford is a registered trade mark of Oxford University Press
in the UK and in certain other countries

Published in the United States
by Oxford University Press Inc., New York

British Library Cataloguing in Publication Data
Data available

Library of Congress Cataloging in Publication Data
Data available

Typeset in GillHandbook by Glyph International, Bangalore, India
Printed and bound by CPI Group (UK) Ltd, Croydon, CR0 4YY

ISBN 978–0–19–957302–8

Acknowledgments

We would like to thank the following for their permissions: Association of Anaesthetists of Great Britain and Ireland; Difficult Airway Society; National Patient Safety Agency; Portex; Resuscitation Council (UK).

Thank you also to: the microbiology and infection control departments at the Royal Berkshire Hospital; Jesse Brown for his great illustrations and patience dealing with us; Mark Bryant, Radiology Specialist Registrar in the Wessex Deanery, for supplying many of the x-ray and ultrasound images; Gary Croucher for his help with photography; all the patients who kindly consented to photography.

GJ, CW, NS

Finally, a big thank you to my wife, Georgia, and my children who put up with me during the hours of writing!

GJ

Contents

Chapter 7 Neurological and Related Procedures 207

Abbreviations

AAGBI – Association of Anaesthetists of Great Britain and Ireland
ANTT – aseptic non-touch technique
ARDS – acute respiratory distress syndrome
ASB – assisted spontaneous breathing
BAL – bronchoalveolar lavage
BiPAP – bi-level positive airway pressure
BP – blood pressure
C-spine – cervical spine
CBF – cerebral blood flow
CMV – controlled mandatory ventilation
CNS – central nervous system
COPD – chronic obstructive pulmonary disease
CPAP – continuous positive airway pressure
CPP – cerebral perfusion pressure
CPR – cardiopulmonary resuscitation
CRRT – continuous renal replacement therapy
CSF – cerebrospinal fluid
CVC – central venous catheter
CVS – cardiovascular system
CVVH – continuous venovenous haemofiltration
CVVHD – continuous venovenous haemodialysis
CVVHDF – continuous venovenous haemodiafiltration
CXR – chest X-ray
DAS – Difficult Airway Society
ECG – electrocardiogram
ENT – ear, nose and throat
ETCO2 – end-tidal carbon dioxide
FRC – functional residual capacity
GCS – Glasgow coma scale
GI – gastrointestinal
HCWs – healthcare workers
HDF – haemodiafiltration
HF – haemofiltration
HFJV – high-frequency jet ventilation
HFO – high-frequency oscillation
ICP – intracranial pressure
LMA – laryngeal mask airway
LP – lumbar puncture
MAP – mean arterial pressure
NG – nasogastric
NICE – National Institute of Clinical Excellence
NIV – non-invasive ventilation

NJ – nasojejunal
PAC – pulmonary artery catheter
PCV – pressure-controlled ventilation
PAoP – pulmonary artery occlusion pressure
PEEP – positive end-expiratory pressure
PICC – peripherally inserted central catheter
PPCD – post-paracentesis circulatory dysfunction
PRAM – pressure recording analytical method
PS – pressure support
RS – respiratory system
RSI – rapid sequence induction
SAH – subarachnoid haemorrhage
SIMV – synchronized intermittent mandatory ventilation
SIRS – systemic inflammatory response syndrome
TIVA – total intravenous anaesthesia
TPN – total parenteral nutrition
TT – tracheal tube
UF – ultrafiltration
USS – ultra-sound scan

Introduction

A book on practical procedures may seem to some superfluous in the era of the Internet, but not to us. A practical procedures book is a familiar friend to be kept at hand; one needs to know the book and where to find the information one wants. As doctors we need to be familiar with a particular approach to a technique. What we do not want to do is to try something new, a variation on a theme, which appeared on the internet, in the early hours of the morning. The ability to perform a wide variety of practical procedures safely and competently is essential for any doctor involved in the practice of anaesthesia and intensive care. Not all of us do all of them regularly, but most of us get called upon to do most of them at some time, often a time not of our choosing. We were taught that one cannot escape statistics and that some procedures carry an intrinsic complication rate but we also believe that attention to detail can keep those complications at the lowest level possible. That is your responsibility to your patients. This book, we hope, will be a helpful companion to those practising procedures and a reassuring safeguard for those undergoing procedures.

The morbidity associated with many procedures may be minimized by ensuring practitioners have familiarity and competence. Historically this has been achieved through long hours at work and learning by example – 'see one, do one, teach one'. However, the reduced hours and changing work patterns of recent times have made the acquisition of practical skills more difficult. In our experience it is still not uncommon for junior anaesthetists and intensivists to be faced with having to perform certain procedures with which they have little familiarity. This is especially true 'out of hours'. One of the authors performed admirably on his first night as a house officer by teaching himself how to record a 12-lead ECG when all around refused to help! It is clear that a book cannot replace practical instruction and formal clinical supervision when it comes to learning practical procedures and none of the techniques described hereafter should be attempted without proper training. However, having a familiar aide-memoire is not only reassuring but also sensible.

To ensure safety, there is no substitute for adequate preparation. Preparation starts with a careful risk/benefit analysis, requires knowledge, which may need refreshing, and needs skill, which implies practice or at least experience. Attention to detail encompasses checking equipment before starting, meticulous attention to cleanliness, and care throughout the performance of a procedure. Post-procedural follow up is also very important and requires a checklist of the potential problems to look out for, a checklist that most of us do not carry, supratentorially, at all times.

We have written this book in the hope that it will be of use to trainees when familiarizing themselves with procedures they are being taught to perform, and also as a reference tool for use at the bedside when performing those procedures alone. We have endeavoured to keep the emphasis on the practical nature of the techniques, hence the use of pictures and illustrations. In addition, we have included many 'handy hints' that

Introduction

we have picked up over the years, which may help others to achieve success with difficult procedures. We cannot take credit for these and therefore send our thanks to all of the wise folk with whom we have worked in the past.

We would welcome your feedback on the book. Please do let us know of any tips or advice you might have for any of the procedures in this book. All comments are gratefully received and can be emailed to us at ost@oup.com.

Guy Jackson
Neil Soni
Chris Whiten
2010

Note:

Please note that some of the photos are intended to demonstrate surface anatomy and have therefore been taken with no attempt to achieve sterility. We promote the highest standards of sterility as demonstrated by our text on the subject.

Chapter 1

Basic Principles

Hand washing

- There has been huge interest in this topic recently, both within medical publications and the media.
- Hands are the most common way in which micro-organisms, particularly bacteria, can be transmitted and subsequently cause infection, especially to those with increased susceptibility. In order to prevent the spread of micro-organisms via this route to those who might develop serious infections while receiving care, hand hygiene must be performed adequately and consistently. This is considered to be the single most important practice in reducing the transmission of infectious agents, and preventing healthcare-associated infections, during delivery of care.
- Every person encountered could be carrying potentially harmful micro-organisms that might be transmitted and cause harm to others. For this reason, hand hygiene is one precaution that must be applied as standard.
- Many hospital trusts now operate a "bare below the elbow" policy following guidance from the Department of Health (Department of Health, 2007).
- The term hand hygiene (decontamination) refers to a process for the physical removal of blood, body fluids and removal or destruction of microorganisms from the hands by hand washing with liquid soap and water and hand decontamination achieved using an alcohol based hand rub.
- Be aware that different techniques may be applicable to different organisms. For example, MRSA requires alcohol-based hand cleaning while *Clostridium difficile* spores need soap and water handwashing.

Definitions

- Social Hand Hygiene
  - This aims to render the hands physically clean and to remove micro-organisms picked up during social activities (transient micro-organisms).
  - Transient flora, which colonize the superficial layers of the skin, are more amenable to removal by routine hand washing. They are often acquired by health care workers (HCWs) during direct contact with patients or contact with contaminated environmental surfaces within close proximity to the patients. Transient flora includes the organisms most frequently associated with healthcare associated infections.
- Hygienic Hand Hygiene
  - Used to remove or destroy transient micro-organisms and to provide residual protection at times when hygiene is particularly important in protecting yourself and others, by reducing resident micro-organisms.
  - Resident flora, which are attached to deeper layers of the skin, are more resistant to removal. In addition, resident flora can cause infections when they are introduced during invasive procedures such as the insertion of intravenous (IV) lines or during surgery.
- Surgical Hand Hygiene
  - Aims to remove or destroy transient micro-organisms and substantially reduce those micro-organisms which normally live on the skin (resident micro-organisms) at times when surgical procedures are being carried out.
  - See 'aseptic technique' section.

Indications

- Before:
  - entering/leaving clinical areas
  - patient contact
  - handling a patient device
  - putting on gloves
  - preparing/giving medications
  - moving from a contaminated body site to a clean body site during patient care
  - using a computer keyboard or mouse (in a clinical area)
  - eating/handling of food/drinks
  - aseptic procedures
  - different care activities for the same patient.
- After:
  - patient contact
  - hands becoming visibly/potentially soiled
  - visiting the toilet
  - using computer keyboard (in a clinical area)
  - handling laundry/equipment/waste
  - blowing/wiping/touching nose
  - any contact with inanimate objects (e.g. equipment, items around the patient) and the patient environment
  - handling body substances
  - **removing gloves**
  - contact with patients being cared for in isolation
  - being in wards during outbreaks of infection.

Contraindications

- None

Complications

- Contact dermatitis

Equipment

- Alcohol based hand gel:
  - must only be used on visibly clean hands. It offers a quick and effective hand decontamination option between care tasks **not** involving body fluids.
- Liquid soap and water:
  - must be used when hands are visibly/potentially soiled with blood or other body fluids.
- Combination of the above:
  - where infection with a spore forming organism e.g. *Clostridium difficile* is suspected/proven.
  - where infection with viral gastroenteritis e.g. Norovirus is suspected.

Sites

- As indicated in Figures 1.1–1.2.
- Commonly missed sites during hand cleaning can be seen in Figure 1.3.

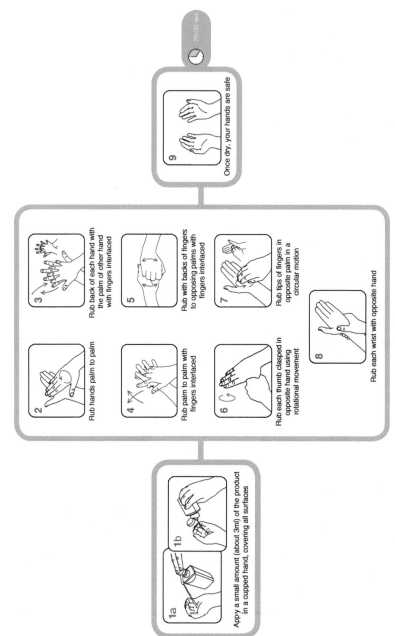

Figure 1.1 How to handwash. Reproduced with kind permission of the National Patient Safety Agency 'cleanyourhands' campaign.

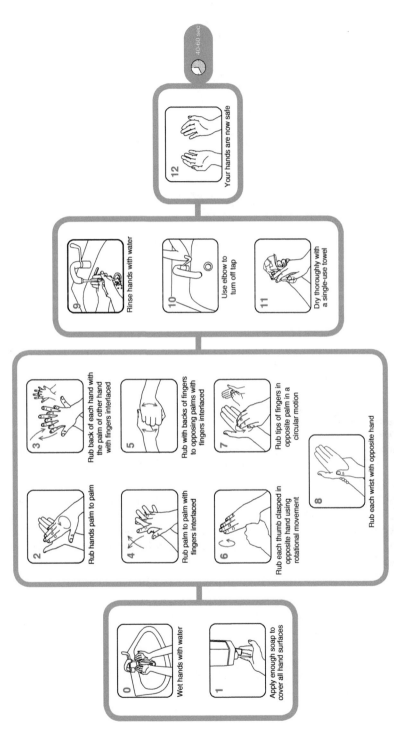

Figure 1.2 How to handrub. Reproduced with kind permission of the National Patient Safety Agency 'cleanyourhands' campaign.

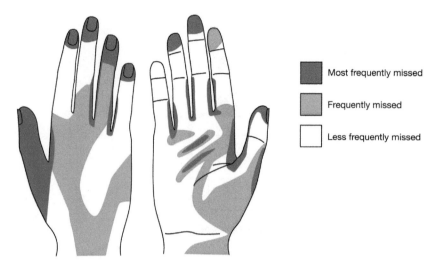

Most frequently missed

Frequently missed

Less frequently missed

Figure 1.3 Commonly missed areas with handwashing (Taylor 1978). With permission from *The Nursing Times*.

Technique

● See Figures 1.1–1.2.

References/further reading

UK Department of Health. (2007). Uniforms and Workwear. *An evidence base for developing local policy.* Available at http://www.dh.gov.uk/

Magos A, Maclean A, Baker D, et al. (2007). "Bare below the elbows"—A cheap soundbite. Letters. *BMJ* 335 p. 684.

Pratt R.J, Pellowe C.M, Wilson J.A et al. (2007). Epic 2: National Evidence Based Guidelines for Preventing Healthcare Associated Infections in NHS Hospitals in England. *Journal of Hospital Infection*, 65 p. S1–S64.

UK National Patient Safety Agency. *'cleanyourhands' campaign.* www.npsa.nhs.uk/cleanyourhands/

Taylor, L. (1978). An evaluation of hand washing techniques -1. *Nursing Times* p.54–55.

Acknowledgements

This section has been written using the guidance contained in the 'Hand Hygiene Protocol' written by Dr N. Virgincar, Consultant Microbiologist and D. Thackray, Infection Control Nurse at the Royal Berkshire Hospital, Royal Berkshire NHS Trust, Reading. We are grateful to the authors of the protocol for allowing us to publish their (abridged) protocol.

Aseptic technique

- Asepsis is the state of being free from all living pathogenic micro-organisms. Aseptic technique refers to a set of specific practices and procedures performed under carefully controlled conditions. These aim to minimize the occurrence of microbial contamination during invasive procedures or when undertaking wound care, and to prevent transmission of pathogenic micro-organisms during patient care.
- Poor aseptic technique can lead to cross-contamination of susceptible patient sites with micro-organisms from the hands of healthcare workers and/or equipment used in treatment, which can result in life threatening infections (Pratt et al. 2007). Aseptic technique should be used during any invasive procedure that bypasses the body's natural defence systems, i.e. the skin or mucous membranes. Aseptic technique serves to maximize and maintain asepsis in order to protect the patient from infection, and to prevent spread/transmission of pathogens to other patients or healthcare workers during patient care.
- Two types of asepsis can be classified:
  - medical/clean asepsis, which aims to reduce the numbers of potentially harmful pathogens and to prevent their spread. It applies to those practices undertaken in clinical areas, but may include treatment areas such as outpatients and primary care clinics.
  - surgical/sterile asepsis, which is a strict process and includes procedures designed to eliminate microorganisms from a site, and generally applies to procedures undertaken in an operating theatre. It is also appropriate on wards and in other departments when invasive procedures (such as insertion of central venous catheters) are performed.
- The procedures are classified as:
  - aseptic non-touch technique (ANTT) using hand decontamination and use of non-sterile gloves.
  - aseptic technique.
  - hand antisepsis (washing/decontamination and appropriate use of gloves).
  - barrier precaution (gloves, aprons, drapes to maintain a sterile field, safe technique, safe environment, e.g. placement of central venous catheters in an operating theatre).
  - skin/mucosal preparation/antisepsis.
  - use and maintenance of sterile patient equipment i.e. sterile/decontaminated instruments/single use devices.

Indications

- Placement of devices or medications into sterile body spaces such as:
  - intravascular catheters, IV lines, central venous catheters (CVCs), vascaths
  - indwelling urinary catheters (urethral, supra-pubic)
  - chest drains
  - ascitic tap/drain
  - insertion of drains into body spaces under radiological guidance
  - lumbar puncture
  - epidurals and spinals.
- Wound care:
  - when dressing wounds that are healing by primary intention e.g. surgical wounds, burns, lacerations including self-harm injuries.

- when dressing wounds that are healing by secondary intention, e.g. pressure sores, leg ulcers, simple grazes.
- when removing drains or sutures from wounds.
- manipulating or dressing an invasive device e.g. cannula, chest drain, urinary catheter.
- taking a sample of urine from an indwelling urinary catheter, accessing a central venous catheter.
- During preparation and administration of intravenous medications via central venous catheters.
- Recommended technique for commonly performed procedures (not an exhaustive list):
  - ANTT: venepuncture, blood culture, intravenous peripheral cannula
  - aseptic: CVC, insertion of chest drain, lumbar puncture, surgical asepsis, urethral catheter insertion.

Contraindications

- Allergy to specific cleaning solution

Equipment

- Running water
- Antiseptic scrub; any of the following:
  - chlorhexidine 4%.
  - povidone-Iodine 7.5% w/w (0.75% w/w available iodine).
  - aqueous alcohol solutions.
  - The choice between of solution is subject to debate and beyond the remit of this book (Tanner et al. 2008).
- Surgical gown
- Sterile gloves
- Theatre hat
- Surgical mask
- Antiseptic solution; any of the following:
  - chlorhexidine based solutions.
  - 0.5% Chlorhexidine in 70% alcohol solution.
  - 2% Chlorhexidine in 70% alcohol solution.
  - iodine based solutions.
  - The choice of solution is subject to debate and beyond the remit of this book.
- Sterile drapes

Technique

- Explain and discuss the procedure with the patient. Gain verbal consent for the procedure.
- Clean dressing trolley using 70% isopropyl alcohol, or, if visibly dirty, with general purpose detergent and water followed by 70% isopropyl alcohol.
- Collect sterile dressing pack and all equipment necessary for procedure. Check packaging is intact and within expiry date and place on bottom of clean trolley.
- Take patient to treatment room if appropriate, or screen bed area. Position patient comfortably so that the area to be treated is easily accessible without excessive exposure. Raise or lower bed to a comfortable working position, and position lighting.

- Perform effective hand decontamination and wash with soap and water.
- Open the outer packing of the dressing pack and tip onto top of trolley.
- Open sterile field using only the corners of the dressing.
- Gently open all other relevant packets, and equipment, and drop onto sterile field.
- Open gown packet, using only the corners, then drop sterile gloves onto this sterile field.
- Apply surgical mask.
- Decontaminate hands by using a 'surgical scrub' technique.
  - Remove all jewellery (rings, watches, bracelets).
  - Wash hands and arms with chlorhexidine or iodine solutions (as above).
  - Clean subungual areas with a nail brush or pick.
  - Scrub each side of each finger, between the fingers, and the back and front of the hand for two minutes.
  - Scrub the arms, keeping the hand higher than the arm at all times. This prevents bacteria-laden soap and water from contaminating the hand.
  - Wash each side of the arm to three inches above the elbow for one minute.
  - Repeat the process on the other hand and arm, keeping hands above elbows at all times.
  - Rinse hands and arms by passing them through the water in one direction only, from fingertips to elbow. Do not move the arm back and forth through the water.
  - Move towards the opened gown and gloves holding hands above elbows.
  - Dry hands and arms using a sterile towel.
  - Apply the gown. It has already been folded so that the outside faces away.
  - Place hands inside the armholes and guide each arm through the sleeves by raising and spreading the arms. Do not allow hands to slide outside the gown cuff.
  - To don gloves, lay the glove palm down over the cuff of the gown. The fingers of the glove face toward you. Working through the gown sleeve, grasp the cuff of the glove and bring it over the open cuff of the sleeve. Unroll the glove cuff so that it covers the sleeve cuff. Proceed with the opposite hand, using the same technique. Never allow the bare hand to contact the gown cuff edge or outside of glove.
- Prepare equipment on the trolley ready for procedure.
- Clean patient's skin using appropriate cleaning solution (as above).
- Using sterile drapes, ideally one with a pre-cut hole, cover any unsterile areas around the site of the cleaned skin. The size of the drape/s should reflect the requirements for the procedure.
  - Some procedures e.g. pulmonary artery catheter insertion, require large drapes for laying out a relatively large amount of equipment.
- At the end of the procedure cover the insertion site with an appropriate sterile dressing.
- Dispose of sharps in a sharps bin and other waste in a yellow plastic clinical waste bag. Remove gown and gloves.
- Clean trolley with water and general purpose detergent and dry thoroughly with paper towel.
- Wash hands with soap and water.

References/further reading

Pratt, R.J. Pellowe, C.M. Wilson et al. (2007). Epic 2: National Evidence-based Guidelines for Preventing Healthcare-Associated Infections in NHS Hospitals in England. *Journal of Hospital Infection*, 65 p. S1–S31.

Tanner J, Swarbrook S, Stuart J. (2008) Surgical hand antisepsis to reduce surgical site infection. *Cochrane Database Syst Rev.* 23, 1:CD004288.

Acknowledgements

This section has been written using the guidance contained in the 'Aseptic Technique Protocol' written by Wendy Morris, Infection Control Nurse, and Shabnam Iyer, Consultant Microbiologist, both at the Royal Berkshire Hospital, Royal Berkshire NHS Trust, Reading. We are grateful to the authors of the protocol for allowing us to publish their (abridged) protocol.

Consent

There has recently been a huge increase in the guidance written on the subject of consent, including exploration of consent in medical practice as a whole, and more specifically within anaesthetic practice. Patient awareness of consent and especially the desire for more information and more choice have dramatically changed.

The General Medical Council introduced updated guidance on 2nd June 2008 (General Medical Council 2008) and the Mental Capacity Act 2005 came into force, in England and Wales, in October 2008. In Scotland there is separate guidance on the capacity to consent contained within the Adults with Incapacity (Scotland) Act 2000.

The Association of Anaesthetists of Great Britain and Ireland have also written guidance on consent for anaesthesia (AAGBI 2006). These documents have clarified much of the thinking about the consent process for doctors and within healthcare as a whole. Inevitably, however, there still remain aspects that are difficult to clarify with generic guidance documents and even by statute law. These issues will continue to be discussed within medical journals and legal circles and will develop over time in response to these, and other, documents.

There are three main components to valid consent.
- Information:
  - the patient must have sufficient information to make a choice.
- Capacity:
  - the patient must be competent.
- Voluntariness:
  - the patient must be able to give their consent freely.

For any practical procedure conducted within anaesthetic practice consent should be sought. This will usually be verbal but in some circumstances this will be written. Documentation of the discussion is vital.

In the event of unexpected procedures, in an emergency setting, patients are often incapacitated and unable to give consent. In this situation we should continue to act in the patient's best interest and carry out any procedure clinically indicated. The AAGBI guidance states that 'if an adult patient is not competent to consent to or refuse treatment (for example, because they are unconscious), immediate treatment that is necessary to preserve the life or health of the patient may be provided in the patient's best interests,' and that 'legally, 'best interests' are more than just 'medical best interests', and include other personal, social and financial factors.'

There should be professional consensus on the need for the procedure. It is wise to discuss what needs to be done, why and what might go wrong, with those who are concerned for the patient (not necessarily next of kin). However, although it is undoubtedly good practice to consult with relatives, no-one can consent to medical, surgical or dental treatment on behalf of an incapable adult patient.

It is good practice to document the reasoning behind any decisions, and any discussions regarding the decision.

References/further reading

Association of Anaesthetists of Great Britain and Ireland (AAGBI) (2006). *Consent in Anaesthesia*.
Scotland. *Adults with Incapacity Act: Elizabeth II* (2000). Available at www.opsi.gov.uk.
General Medical Council (2008). *Consent: patients and doctors making decisions together*.
UK. *Mental Capacity Act Chapter 9: Elizabeth II* (2005). Available at www.opsi.gov.uk

Environment, safety and additional equipment

All invasive procedures are associated with risk to the patient (and potentially to the practitioner). In order to reduce these risks, or at least to be able to deal with them should the need arise, procedures should be carried out in an environment with access to appropriate equipment, facilities and staff. Many would agree, especially anaesthetists, that the best environment for most procedures would be an anaesthetic room or the operating room itself. Obviously this is not always possible, for instance patients may be too unstable, clinically, to transfer to such an area. Often these procedures will be carried out on intensive care units or emergency departments where it remains essential to maintain adequate equipment, facilities and staffing in order to maximize safety, thereby maximizing the chances of a successful procedure.

To this end it is also important to understand the intended procedure, including the indications, complications and procedural elements themselves.

A method for describing any procedure can be remembered by using the following mnemonic. As well as being useful for answering questions on any procedure for postgraduate exams, it is also useful to ensure adequate preparation before commencing any procedure. Adequate preparation goes a long way towards achieving success with practical procedures.

I Can Pull Pretty Ladies (or Lads!) eSpecially Charlie

- **I**ndications:
  - as detailed in each section later.
- **C**ontraindications:
  - as detailed in each section later.
- **P**reparation:
  - safe environment e.g. anaesthetic room
  - tilting trolley
  - oxygen
  - suction
  - monitoring
  - trained assistant
  - equipment for specific procedure
  - emergency drugs
  - emergency equipment
  - resuscitation facilities.
- **P**rocedure:
  - as detailed in each section later.
- **L**andmarks:
  - as detailed in each section later.
- **S**olution (if injecting any local anaesthetic e.g. regional nerve blocks).
- **C**omplications:
  - as detailed in each section later.

Acknowledgements

Thanks to Dr D. Smith, Consultant Anaesthetist, The Hillingdon Hospital for teaching the author (GJ) this mnemonic.

Ultrasound in anaesthesia and intensive care

- The use of ultrasound as an aid in a number of practical procedures is becoming more and more widespread. This can either be in 'real time' (such as for central line insertion when the probe is held to the skin during the needle insertion) or for marking the site of insertion (e.g. for locating a pleural infusion prior to Seldinger chest drain insertion).

Indications

Common:
- internal jugular CVC
- femoral CVC
- Seldinger chest drain insertion
- Ultrasound-guided nerve blockade and regional anaesthesia.

Uncommon:
- subclavian CVC (difficult to visualize)
- arterial line insertion.

Contraindications

- None.

Complications

- None directly due to the ultrasound probe or wave.
- Indirectly the ultrasound and the picture produced can be the source of distraction and if employed without understanding of the principles involved can be used in a dangerous manner. It is important to understand that the picture displayed on the screen is a 2D, not a 3D image. Therefore the image shown is simply a slice through an anatomical plane.
- The physical landmarks are still important, as is the pulsatility of the visualized vessel.
  - Physical examination always complement ultrasound.
  - In a hypovolaemic hypotensive patient a barely pulsatile and collapsible carotid artery can be mistaken for a vein.

Equipment

- Ultrasound machine
- Sterile probe cover/sheath
- Sterile lubricating gel

Sites

- Suitable for jugular and femoral CVC insertions.
- Can also be used to visualize arteries and peripheral veins.
- Less useful for subclavian CVC insertion.
- Any accessible peripheral nerve.

Insertion

- See section on CVC insertion using ultrasound (USS) section.

Tips and advice

- There are many makes and models of ultrasound machines available. There is no substitute for familiarizing oneself with the model available locally before use in clinical practice. Particular note should be made of how to adjust the depth of the signal (i.e. the penetration of the image displayed), how to measure distances on the monitor and how to adjust the contrast.

Cardiopulmonary resuscitation

- The Resuscitation Council (UK) was formed in August 1981 by a group of medical practitioners from a variety of specialities who shared an interest in, and concern for, the subject of resuscitation.
- Working Parties of the Resuscitation Council (UK) regularly review the protocols for basic, advanced, paediatric, and newborn resuscitation. The guidelines accompanying this section are reproduced with the kind permission of the Resuscitation Council (UK).
- Detailed discussion of all resuscitation guidance is beyond the remit of this book and readers are directed towards the resuscitation departments within their own hospitals and the national and international organisations along with their affiliated training programmes.

Technique

- Figures 1.4–1.7 show the algorithms for adult advanced life support, paediatric advanced life support, and the management of adult tachycardic and bradycardic rhythms.
- Figures 1.8–1.10 demonstrate some of the procedural elements of the resuscitation process including precordial thump, hand positioning for undertaking cardiac compressions and correct positioning of defibrillator pads.

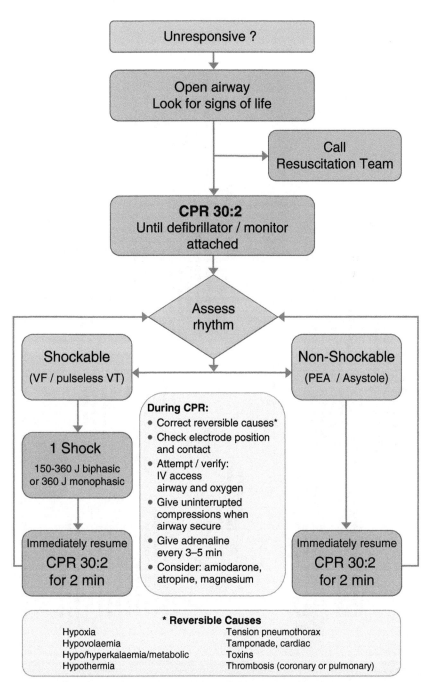

Figure 1.4 Adult Advanced Life Support algorithm. Reproduced with the kind permission of the Resuscitation Council (UK).

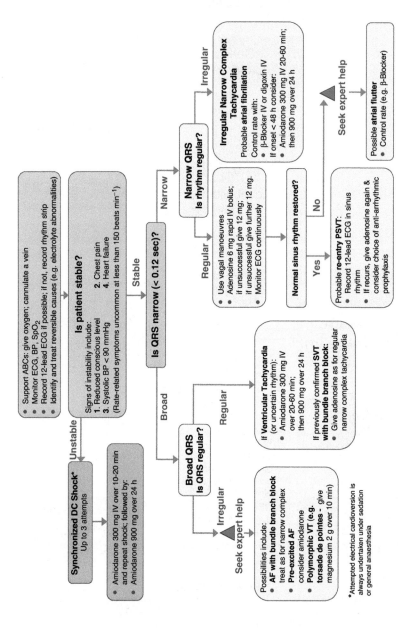

Figure 1.5 Adult tachycardia algorithm. Reproduced with the kind permission of the Resuscitation Council (UK).

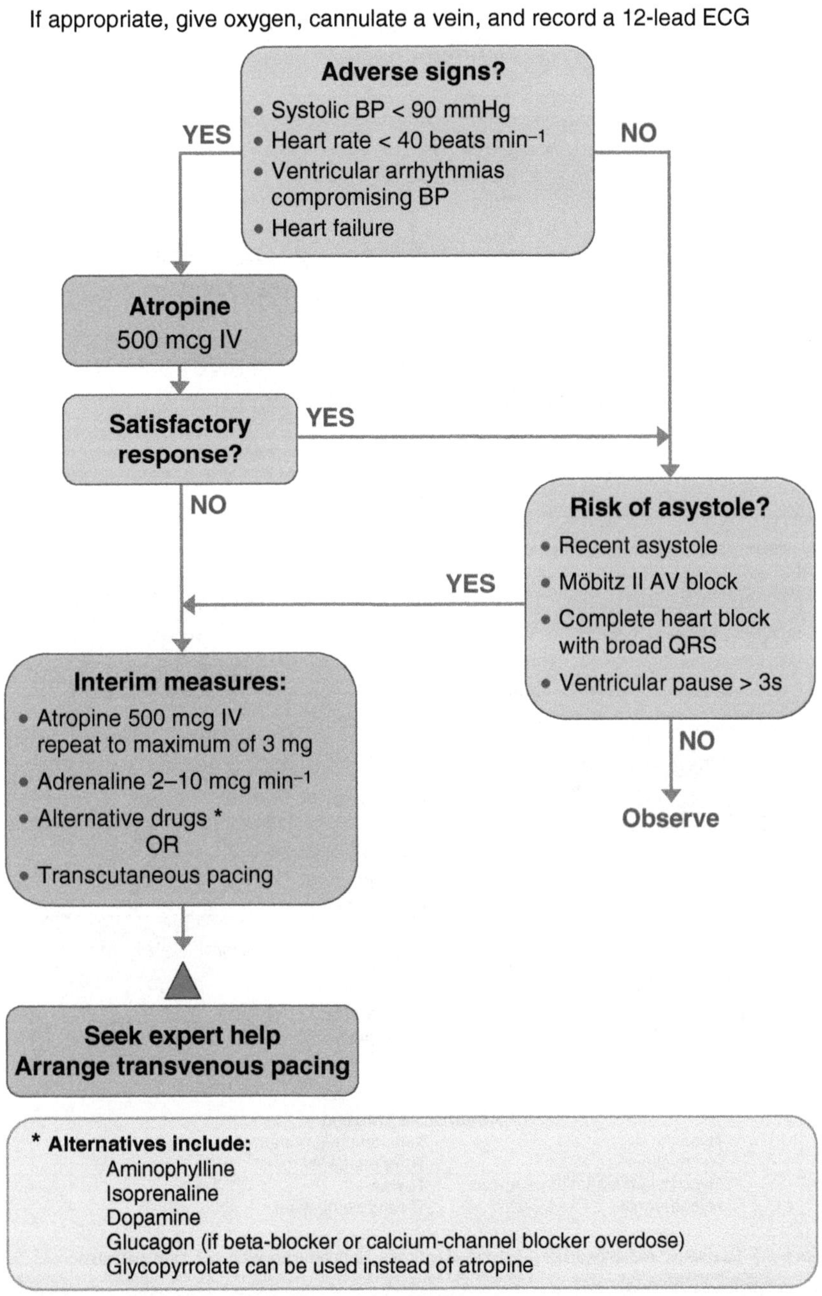

If appropriate, give oxygen, cannulate a vein, and record a 12-lead ECG

Adverse signs?

- Systolic BP < 90 mmHg
- Heart rate < 40 beats min^{-1}
- Ventricular arrhythmias compromising BP
- Heart failure

YES / NO

Atropine
500 mcg IV

Satisfactory response? — YES

NO

Risk of asystole?

- Recent asystole
- Möbitz II AV block
- Complete heart block with broad QRS
- Ventricular pause > 3s

YES

NO

Interim measures:

- Atropine 500 mcg IV repeat to maximum of 3 mg
- Adrenaline 2–10 mcg min^{-1}
- Alternative drugs *
  OR
- Transcutaneous pacing

Observe

Seek expert help
Arrange transvenous pacing

> *** Alternatives include:**
> Aminophylline
> Isoprenaline
> Dopamine
> Glucagon (if beta-blocker or calcium-channel blocker overdose)
> Glycopyrrolate can be used instead of atropine

Figure 1.6 ALS Adult bradycardia algorithm. Reproduced with the kind permission of the Resuscitation Council (UK).

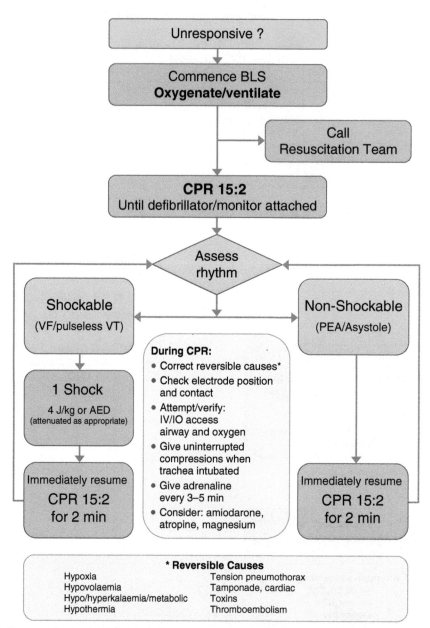

Figure 1.7 Paediatric Advanced Life Support algorithm. Reproduced with the kind permission of the Resuscitation Council (UK).

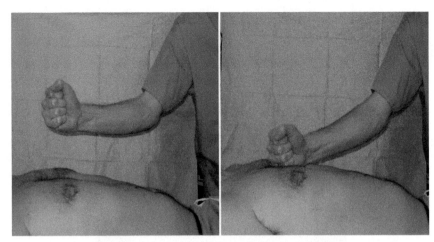

Figure 1.8 Precordial thump.

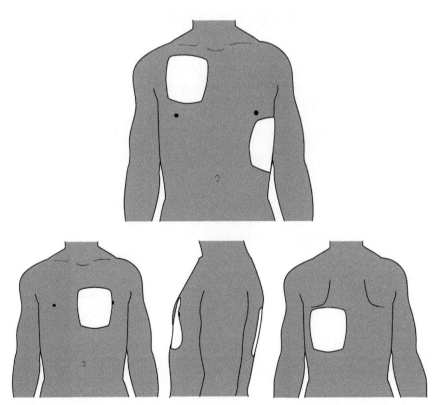

Figure 1.9 Positioning of adhesive pads for defibrillation.

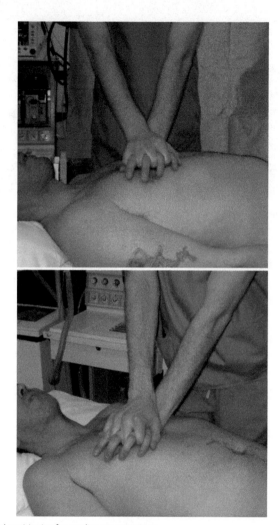

Figure 1.10 Hand positioning for cardiac compressions.

References/further reading

Resuscitation Council (UK). *Advanced Life Support. 5th Edition.* (2006). www.resus.org.uk

Chapter 2

Intravascular Access

Peripheral venous cannulation

Indications

- Administration of drugs and fluids
- Venesection

Contraindications

- Absolute:
  - none.
- Relative:
  - coagulopathy
  - skin/soft-tissue infections at site

Complications

- Failure to cannulate
  - Limit to 2 attempts, then summon help
- Haematoma formation/bleeding
  - Apply pressure
- Thrombosis
- Infection
  - Risk increased after cannula in situ for greater than 48 hours
- Inflammation
  - Especially when irritant substances injected
- Accidental arterial cannulation

Equipment

- Many hospitals now have intravenous cannula packs containing all the equipment required to place a cannula using an aseptic technique. If such a pack is not available the following are required:
  - antiseptic
  - gauze (sterile)
  - local anaesthetic (topical or subcutaneous); generally used for >20G cannulae in adults (see local anaesthesia chapter)
  - sterile saline flush
  - polyurethane cannula (older versions are PVC) with 'flashback chamber.'
    - Gauge determines flow rate (see Table 2.1; Yentis 2000).
    - Smaller gauge equals lower risk of phlebitis.
    - Use smallest gauge for prescribed therapy:
      - 14–16G for resuscitation
      - 20–22G for maintenance fluids.
  - sterile moisture-permeable transparent dressing.

Table 2.1 Flow rates dependent on gauge; Yentis (2000)

Gauge	Flow rate ml/min
20G	40–80
18G	75–120
16G	130–220
14G	250–360

Table 2.2 Colour coding for IV cannulae

Gauge	Colour
24G	Yellow
22G	Blue
20G	Pink
18G	Green
17G	White
16G	Grey
14G	Orange

Sites

- Multiple insertion sites usable:
  - hand and arm most common.
  - foot and leg:
    - limits mobility
    - thrombosis risk.
- Start distally and work proximally if attempt fails:
  - prevents leakage of fluid from failure site.
- Avoid sites over joints/close to arteries.
- Remember patient comfort:
  - antecubital fossa often uncomfortable and cannula can occlude with flexion of elbow.
- Basilic vein on forearm often overlooked:
  - can be useful in difficult cases.

Insertion

- Apply tourniquet proximal to chosen insertion site.
- Clean the area around the chosen vein and, ideally, use a sterile drape (dependent on degree of urgency).
- Infiltrate local anaesthetic (if required) overlying, or just lateral to, vein.
- Hold the cannula either:
  - with hub between thumb and forefinger, or
  - with thumb on cap and forefinger and/or middle finger supporting the hub (see Figures 2.1 and 2.2).
- Support and stabilize the patient's hand (resting on pillow works well).
- Stretch the surrounding skin to minimize movement of skin on needle insertion.
- Penetrate skin through anaesthetized area, aiming towards vein.
- Advance needle towards vein until hub fills with blood.
- Ensure cannula, not just tip of needle, is in the vein.
- Advance cannula over needle until hub at skin.
- Remove tourniquet.
- Withdraw needle.
- Attach syringe for blood collection if required (may require tourniquet to ensure adequate filling of vein to allow blood aspiration).
- Attach cap or fluid line as required.
- Secure firmly in place using a sterile dressing.

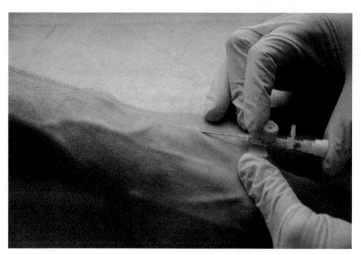

Figure 2.1 Peripheral venous cannulation demonstrating different methods of holding the cannula. One method of holding the cannula. Note the skin tension, stabilising the skin and underlying vein, using the left thumb.

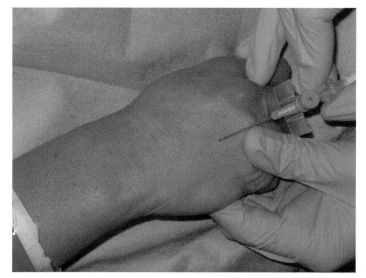

Figure 2.2 Peripheral venous cannulation demonstrating different methods of holding the cannula. Alternative method of holding cannula.

Important points/cautions

- The tip of the needle can protrude a significant distance from the cannula. If the needle is only advanced a short distance into the vein it is then common to have problems advancing the cannula over the needle (especially with larger cannulae). Look at some cannulae to get an idea of how far the needles protrude (note variations between manufacturers).

Tips and advice

- Ensure that you are positioned comfortably. It is far easier to cannulate successfully if sitting down in a comfortable position with a well-positioned vein.

- If possible, take time to optimize the appearance of the vein with adequate venous stasis and gentle massage, or tapping, over the area to encourage venous dilation. This aids both visualization and consequently successful cannulation.
- Make efforts to 'fix' the chosen vein. A mobile vein is difficult to cannulate.
- It often requires considerable force to advance the needle through the skin. This can be aided by approaching the vein from the side and at a steeper angle rather than above and at a shallow angle. One can then re-angle the needle towards the vein at a shallower angle once through the skin.
- If you go through the back of the vein try withdrawing the needle slightly (into the cannula) and then slowly withdrawing the cannula. If the cannula and hub suddenly fill with blood try advancing the cannula as it will now be in the vein.
- Following a failed cannulation, with penetration of the vein, maintain pressure on the vein with gauze after releasing the tourniquet, before attempting cannulation again. This will reduce the risk of haematoma formation.

References/further reading

Yentis SM (2000). In: Yentis S (ed.) *Anaesthesia and Intensive Care A-Z: an encyclopaedia of principles and practice*. p 299. Butterworth-Heinemann, Edinburgh.

Central venous access

Indications

- Measurement
  - Invasive haemodynamic monitoring:
    - central venous pressure
    - pulmonary artery catheters
- Infusion of fluids
- Infusion of drugs
  - Irritant substances:
    - amiodarone, total parenteral nutrition (TPN), inotropes
- Accessing the heart:
  - pacing wire
- Rapid volume infusion:
  - e.g. pulmonary artery introducer sheath
- Difficult peripheral venous access:
  - emergency setting when peripherally 'shut down'
  - electively when peripheral access impossible
    - e.g. intravenous drug users
- Long term venous access:
  - chemotherapy
  - TPN
- Special procedures:
  - renal replacement therapy
  - exchange transfusion
- Aspiration of air from the heart:
  - air emboli

Contraindications

- Absolute:
  - vein thrombosed and occluded (if assessed with ultrasound)
- Relative:
  - patient refusal
  - local sepsis or injury e.g. burns
  - coagulopathy
  - pneumothorax on contralateral side
    - due to potential for bilateral pneumothoraces

Complications

- Common:
  - haemorrhage
  - haematoma formation
  - arterial puncture
  - cardiac dysrhythmias
  - pneumothorax
  - infection
  - venous thrombosis

- Rare:
  - air embolism
  - haemothorax
  - chylothorax
  - neurapraxia
  - cardiac tamponade
  - thoracic duct injury

Equipment

- Tilting bed/trolley
- Portable ultrasound with sterile lubrication gel and sterile sheath
- Sterile pack:
  - Many hospitals now use 'central line' packs that will contain much of the equipment listed below.
- Antiseptic solution
- Local anaesthetic (1% or 2% lidocaine)
- Central venous catheter appropriate for intended use:
  - 1, 2, 3, 4 or 5 lumen
  - sheaths for insertion of pacing wires or pulmonary artery catheter
  - 12F double lumen catheters used for venovenous filtration/dialysis ('Vascaths')
  - single lumen, large bore (14 or 16G), long catheters (usually only used in the emergency setting for central access; non-Seldinger).
- Pressure transducer (set up, ready for use, with fluid infusion system):
  - fine bore extension tubing for confirmation of correct placement (see below)
- Saline or heparinized saline for flushing lines
- Securing device (various available commercially) or suture on a straight needle:
  - non-absorbable 2/0 commonly used.
- Sterile semi-permeable adhesive dressing

Sites

- Internal jugular vein
- Subclavian vein
- Femoral vein

Insertion technique

- See individual approaches and generic technique below.

Generic technique

- Fully explain the procedure to the patient and gain consent.
- If the patient is conscious, explain that their face will be covered by a drape and that they must not touch this sterile area. Reassure the patient that they can still communicate by talking.
- Assistance must be immediately available:
  - no matter how well prepared one is, it is not uncommon to forget items, and once gowned, it is impossible to obtain them without compromising sterility.
- Prepare the patient:
  - sedation if required
  - position appropriately

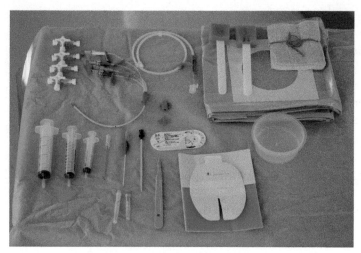

Figure 2.3 CVC equipment preparation: laying up the trolley.

- ○ oxygen mask
- ○ monitoring – pulse oximetry, electrocardiogram (ECG), non-invasive blood pressure as a minimum (See Box 3.1, Recommendations for standards of monitoring during anaesthesia and recovery).
- ● Prepare the equipment:
  - ○ think through the steps involved and ensure all equipment required is available and to hand (See Figure 2.3).
- ● Full aseptic technique – **important!**
- ● Open the equipment and prepare it. Flush all ports with 0.9% saline and lock them.
- ● Clean the skin with antiseptic solution.
- ● Prepare sterile field with drape:
  - ○ ideally, use a large transparent drape with fenestration in centre.
- ● If conscious, infiltrate skin with local anaesthetic (see local anaesthetic chapter).
  - ○ Massage area to avoid distortion of anatomy.
- ● Using either a needle or cannula-over-needle with a 5 or 10 ml syringe attached, locate vein.
  - ○ Aspirate with the syringe gently while advancing needle and ensure easy aspiration of blood.
  - ○ If using cannula-over-needle, then cannulate the vein by sliding the cannula over the needle and into the vein.
- ● Confirm venous placement.
  - ○ Colour (unreliable):
    - ▪ venous blood is darker red in colour.
  - ○ Pressure:
    - ▪ transduce using fine bore extension connected to needle hub and handed to assistant to connect to transducer.
  - ○ Check blood gas sample against arterial sample (time consuming).
- ● Insert guidewire to 15-20 cm.
  - ○ Inserting further risks irritating the myocardium and causing arrhythmias.
  - ○ Watch (or have assistant watch) ECG trace.

- Remove needle, or cannula, over the wire.
  - Ensure wire remains at same depth and does not come out with needle.
- Pass dilator over wire and insert into vein.
  - A small, superficial cut in the skin with a scalpel at the entry point aids insertion of the dilator through the skin.
  - Think of the depth to the vein:
    - the dilator rarely needs to be inserted to the hub and doing so may cause damage.
- Remove dilator over wire, whilst applying slight pressure with gauze over site to reduce bleeding.
  - Level bed (if head down) to reduce bleeding from site if required.
- Thread catheter over wire, whilst ensuring that the proximal end of the wire is in sight at all times to prevent loss of wire in vein.
- Insert the catheter an appropriate distance into patient dependent on site (see individual techniques).
  - Rarely is there a need to insert the catheter deeper than 15 cm (at the skin).
- Confirm venous placement.
- Aspirate blood from every lumen, flush with 0.9% Saline and close and cover all ports.
- Suture catheter to skin.
  - 4-point fixation is ideal to prevent accidental removal or withdrawal of catheter.
  - It also allows withdrawal of the catheter later (under sterile conditions) should the catheter be found to be positioned incorrectly on imaging.
- Cover with sterile transparent semi-permeable dressing.
- Request a chest X-ray (CXR) if required.
- Document procedure in patient's notes.

Technique if two catheters are being placed at the same site

- Insert first guidewire into selected vein as before. Remove needle (or cannula).
- Insert second guidewire into same vein with skin puncture about 0.5–1 cm away from first site. Remove needle (or cannula).
- If two differently sized catheters being placed (e.g. central venous catheter and vascath) then insert smaller catheter at lower insertion site and then larger (stiffer) catheter at higher puncture site.
- **Remember** to note which wire belongs to which catheter as they may be of different lengths/gauges depending on the catheters being placed.

Important points/cautions

- Beware air entrainment, even if patient's head is down.
- Never use excessive force when inserting a wire or catheter.
- Always think of where the needle point is, especially when using ultrasound to guide placement.
- Never lose sight (or hold) of the proximal end of the wire.
  - Wires have been 'lost' inside patients.
- If withdrawing the wire through needle be aware that ANY resistance may result in damage to and/or shearing of the wire.
  - If this occurs withdraw both wire and needle together.

Tips and advice

- Use of pre-packed kits ensures all equipment is immediately available and improves sterile technique.
- If the wire is not advancing easily try changing the direction of the needle slightly, to (usually) a less acute angle, and attempt advancement again.
  - With internal jugular lines, an alternative technique is to have an assistant pull on the patient's **ipsilateral** arm, parallel with their body, in a caudal direction, and then to attempt advancement of the wire again.
- Ensure 'beep volume' for the ECG is clearly audible, to aid recognition of arrhythmias during wire insertion.

Ultrasound guidance for intravenous central line insertion

- Recent studies have demonstrated a reduced complication rate during certain procedures using ultrasound guidance (Wigmore et al. 2007).
- The National Institute of Clinical Excellence (NICE) have produced recommendations entitled 'Guidance on the use of ultrasound locating devices for placing central venous catheters' (NICE 2002) on the use of ultrasound during internal jugular cannulation.
- The NICE guidance is summarized below.
  - Two-dimensional (2D) imaging ultrasound guidance is recommended as the preferred method for insertion of CVCs into the internal jugular vein in adults and children in elective situations.
  - The use of 2D imaging ultrasound guidance should be considered in most clinical circumstances where CVC insertion is necessary either electively or in an emergency situation.
  - It is recommended that all those involved in placing CVCs using 2D imaging ultrasound guidance should undertake appropriate training to achieve competence.

Indications

Common:

- internal jugular CVC insertion
- femoral CVC insertion
- USS is particularly useful in the morbidly obese.

Uncommon:

- subclavian CVC
- external jugular lines.

Contraindications

- None.

Complications

- None due directly to the ultrasound probe or wave.
- Indirectly the ultrasound and the picture produced can be a source of distraction and if used without understanding of the principles can be dangerous. It is important to understand that the picture displayed on the screen is a 2D image, not a 3D image. Therefore the image displayed is simply a slice through an anatomical plane. If that slice is at 90 degrees to the advancing needle then the needle will not be seen to advance in real time, rather to pass through a particular point (slice) at some point on its path. This can sometimes lead to false reassurance that the needle tip is

in sight on the ultrasound display when in fact it is displaying the needle passing through the anatomical slice and the needle tip is somewhere distal. If focus remains on the ultrasound image rather than what the hands and the needle tip are actually doing then inadvertent damage can occur to other vessels, nerves and viscera. It is possible, in skilled hands, to turn the probe to produce a longitudinal anatomical slice which, if placed accurately, can show the advancement of a needle. However this method is not free from the problems described above, and again has the potential to falsely reassure.

Equipment

- Ultrasound machine with linear probe (high frequency 7–12 MHz)
- Sterile probe cover/sheath
- Sterile lubricating gel

Sites

- As above.

Technique

- Prepare the patient for CVC insertion (see earlier section).
- Cover the probe in a sterile manner.
- Use the ultrasound to:
  - ensure normal anatomy exists and aid location of the vein before starting procedure, and/or:
  - in 'real time,' watch the needle tip penetrating the vein. The wire is then inserted in the normal manner before confirming correct placement in the vein, also with ultrasound. USS can also be used to demonstrate the smooth movement of the wire within the vein before dilation for CVC insertion.
- If using the ultrasound in 'real time' there are two methods of holding the probe (see Figure 2.6).
  - Transverse view
  - Longitudinal view
  - Whichever view is used the angle of needle penetration should be altered to enter the vein within view of the 2D image.
- Identify the anatomy using the ultrasound probe, noting patency and depth of vein.
  - See Figure 2.5 for internal jugular anatomy.
  - See Figure 2.4 for femoral anatomy.
- A 45-degree angle of approach towards the vein is best (see Figure 2.6). Whilst watching the ultrasound screen insert needle 1–2 cm (depending on depth of vein) from ultrasound probe.
- Advance needle whilst watching the screen for the appearance of the needle in the 2D image.
- As you press the needle onto the outer wall of the vein it is pushed away to start with, then when the wall gives, the vessel pops over the needle.
  - If the approach is too vertical you run the risk of impaling the posterior wall too.
  - The angle also greatly helps the passing of the guide wire for the same reason. If too vertical it can buckle against the back wall, or even go the wrong way. The distance the needle starts away from the probe all depends on the depth of the structure you are aiming at from the skin surface. Sometimes you have to start further away so that the angle you want to take will take you into the vessel.
- Once the needle is seen within the lumen of the vessel it should be possible to aspirate blood.

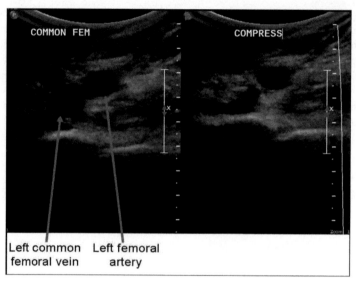

Figure 2.4 USS (transverse) view of left common femoral vein.

- Insert the guidewire and remove the introducer needle.
- Visualize the guidewire within the lumen of the vessel **before** inserting the dilator over the guidewire.
- Proceed as for normal CVC insertion.

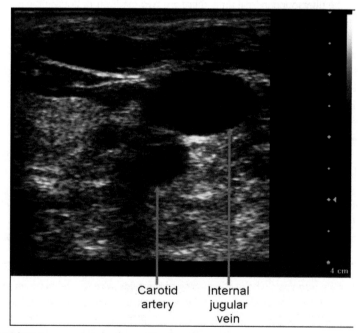

Figure 2.5 USS (transverse) view of internal jugular vein.

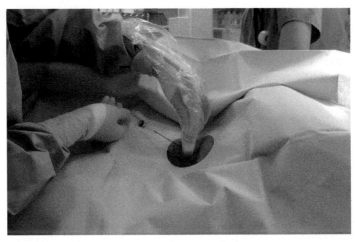

Figure 2.6 Photo demonstrating how to hold probe and needle direction.

Important points/cautions

- It is important to maintain sterile conditions while using ultrasound. This can be achieved by using sheaths to cover the probe and most of the cable leading to the monitor.

Tips and advice

- There are many makes and models of ultrasound machines available. There is no substitute for familiarizing oneself with the model available locally before use in clinical practice. Particular note should be made of how to adjust the depth of the signal (i.e. the penetration of the image displayed), how to measure distances on the monitor and how to adjust the contrast.
- Adjust the depth of the image to obtain the clearest image possible before proceeding with 'real time' insertion.
- Ask an assistant to hold the ultrasound probe (ensuring sterility) in order to free up both hands of the operator.
- If the specific probe cover (sheath) is not available then there are other methods of covering the probe, although sterility will be harder to maintain and they are therefore not recommended.
- Remember to lubricate the probe with jelly prior to covering.

References/further reading

Wigmore TJ, Smythe JF, Hacking MB, Raobaikady R and MacCallum NS (2007). Effect of the implementation of NICE guidelines for ultrasound guidance on the complication rates associated with central venous catheter placement in patients presenting for routine surgery in a tertiary referral centre. *British Journal of Anaesthesia*, 99: 662–665.

UK National Institute of Clinical Excellence (2002). *Central venous catheters - ultrasound locating devices (TA49)*. http://guidance.nice.org.uk/TA49

Seldinger technique

- The Seldinger technique is named after Dr. Sven-Ivar Seldinger (1921–1998), a Swedish radiologist, who introduced the procedure in 1953 (Seldinger 1953).
- It describes a method of using a needle to locate a desired anatomical space (e.g. a blood vessel or body cavity) followed by the insertion of a blunt tipped wire

through the needle . The needle is then removed and the passage dilated in order to allow the passing, over the wire, of a larger cannula or catheter. The wire is then removed.

- It can also be used to replace a catheter already in situ with a different one, using the wire to maintain patency of the passage ('railroading').

Indications

- CVC insertion or replacement*
- Arterial line insertion or replacement*
- Percutaneous chest drain insertion
* See next section.

Contraindications (specific to the Seldinger technique)

- Absolute:
  - vein thrombosed and occluded (if assessed by ultrasound).
- Relative:
  - local sepsis or injury e.g. burns
  - coagulopathy.

Complications (specific to the Seldinger technique)

- Common:
  - difficulty inserting the wire due to misplacement of needle or anatomical abnormalities
  - arterial puncture
  - cardiac dysrhythmias (due to myocardial irritation by wire).
- Rare:
  - air embolism
  - haemothorax
  - neurapraxia
  - cardiac tamponade.

Equipment

- As for generic CVC insertion.
- Introducer needle.
- Seldinger wire: should be soft tipped at one end, and is often J shaped to aid manipulation around corners.
  - These wires are provided within equipment packs, but individually packaged wires are available should there be problems with the first wire used.
- Dilator (appropriately sized for the catheter to be inserted).
- Catheter.

Sites

- Veins: as for generic CVC insertion
- Arteries: as for arterial line insertion
- Chest drains: as marked, prior to insertion, after using ultrasound

Insertion technique

- Full aseptic technique – **important**!
- Open the equipment and prepare. Flush all ports with 0.9% saline and lock.
- Clean the skin with antiseptic.

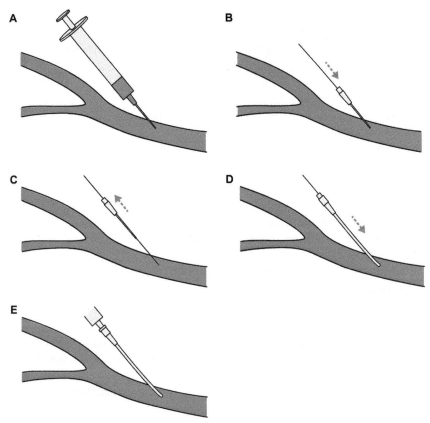

Figure 2.7 Seldinger technique. a. Insert needle (or cannula over needle) into vein, confirming easy aspiration of blood into syringe. Remove needle, if cannula used, covering end of cannula with thumb. b. Insert guidewire into vein via needle (or cannula). c. Remove needle (or catheter) leaving the wire in place. d. Insert dilator. Then remove dilator remembering to apply pressure to insertion site to prevent bleeding on withdrawal of dilator. e. Insert catheter and remove guidewire.

- Prepare sterile field with drape.
  - Ideally large transparent drape with central fenestration.
- If conscious, infiltrate skin with local anaesthetic (see 'local anaesthetic' section).
  - Massage area to avoid distortion of anatomy.
- Using needle or cannula-over-needle (for CVC only) locate vessel.
  - Aspirate gently using a 5 or 10ml syringe (attached to the needle or cannula-over-needle) while advancing and ensure easy aspiration of blood.
- Confirm appropriate placement.
  - Blood (artery or vein):
    - colour (unreliable)
    - pressure
      - arterial placement is usually obvious due to the presence of pulsatile blood.
    - check blood gas sample against arterial sample (time consuming).
  - Pleural fluid or air:
    - if inserting chest drain.

- Insert guidewire.
- Remove needle (or cannula) over guidewire.
  - Ensure wire remains at same depth and does not come out with needle.
- Pass dilator (**not** with arterial lines) over wire and insert into vein.
- Remove dilator (not with arterial lines), whilst applying slight pressure with gauze over site to reduce bleeding.
- Thread catheter over wire ensuring that the end of the wire is in sight at all times to prevent loss of wire in vessel.
- Insert catheter to appropriate depth.
- Ensure correct placement.
- See sections on each technique.

Important points/cautions

- Insert the wire 'floppy end' first (CVC lines).
- The wire must never be inserted 'hard end' first.
- Wires must never be forced.
- Always keep the wire in sight at all times.
  - It is possible to lose the wire into the vein or artery.
- A dilator is only used for insertion of CVCs and chest drains.
- Use care when inserting the dilator.
  - Dilators rarely need to be inserted to the hilt and one should take account of the depth of the vein, to avoid excessive dilator insertion and consequent risk of distal vein perforation.
- Avoid air entrainment on removal of the wire by covering the lumen of the catheter inserted.

References/further reading

Seldinger SI (1953). Catheter replacement of the needle in percutaneous arteriography; a new technique. *Acta radiologica* 39 p. 368–76.

Railroading

- CVC catheters and arterial lines should not routinely be exchanged/replaced using the Seldinger technique due to the inherent increased risk of catheter infection.
- This is not a 'sterile' technique and should only be used in certain circumstances where the anticipated problems of inserting a fresh catheter outweigh the increased risk of line infection with railroading.

Indications

- CVC replacement*
- Arterial line replacement*

When there is a need to replace a line, but there are:

- high risks of complications with a new puncture (e.g. coagulopathy)
- no other sites available.

Contraindications

Absolute:

- known or suspected catheter infection.

Relative:

- coagulopathy

- alternative site available, and no specific contraindications to standard Seldinger CVC insertion technique.

Complications

- Catheter related infections
- Reintroduction of infection
- Bleeding
- Kinking of wire:
  - may lead to problems removing old wire, or inserting new one.

Equipment

- Sterile drapes
- Antiseptic solution
- New CVC
- Syringes
- 0.9% saline
- Three-way taps
- Scalpel
- Skin suture
- Sterile dressing

Sites

- Venous:
  - internal jugular
  - subclavian
  - femoral
- Arterial:
  - radial
  - brachial
  - femoral

Insertion technique

- Full aseptic technique – **important**!
  - It is, however, impossible to maintain full asepsis due to the presence of the line already in situ. Use antiseptic solution to clean the line as much as possible before gowning.
- Open the equipment and prepare.
  - Flush all ports with 0.9% saline and lock.
- Clean the skin with antiseptic solution.
- Prepare sterile field with drape.
- If patient is conscious, infiltrate skin with local anaesthetic (see 'Local anaesthetic' section).
- Insert wire into **distal** port if multilumen catheter.
  - Usually brown port on CVCs, but confirm before insertion.
- Withdraw catheter over wire ensuring wire is always visible and is not pulled out of vessel completely.
- Thread new catheter over wire ensuring that the end of the wire is in sight at all times to prevent loss of wire in vessel.

- Insert catheter to appropriate depth.
- Suture catheter to skin and apply a clean, sterile dressing.
- Ensure correct placement.
  - CXR if appropriate.

Important points/cautions

- Never lose sight of the wire.

Tips and advice

- Once the old catheter is removed ensure wire will advance into the vessel.
  - Ensures wire has not migrated out of the vessel.
- Ensure any drug infusions via CVCs have been discontinued. This technique cannot be used if important drugs, such as inotropes, are being infused at the time!

Internal jugular vein CVC insertion

Indications

- As for generic CVC insertion.
- Compared with the subclavian route:
  - lower incidence of pneumothorax.
    - Preferred in the obese or those with respiratory disease/compromise.
- Compared to the femoral route:
  - more convenient for the anaesthetist in theatre
  - lower incidence of line infection.

Contraindications

- As for generic CVC insertion.
- In presence of raised intracranial pressure (ICP).
  - May reduce venous drainage from the head.

Complications

- As for generic CVC insertion.
- Misplacement in subclavian vein (catheter tip aimed towards arm).
- Arterial puncture is still common even with ultrasound.
- The dome of the lung is within range of the tip of the needle.
- Later complication: thrombosis.

Equipment

- As for generic CVC insertion.

Sites

- Right internal jugular vein:
  - most commonly used.
- Left internal jugular vein:
  - potential for damage to the thoracic duct (only present on the left).
  - often more difficult to insert due to anatomy of veins.

Insertion technique

- As for generic CVC insertion with the addition of the following points:
  - Prepare patient with slight Trendelenburg (head down) position.
  - Remove pillow if required to improve neck extension.

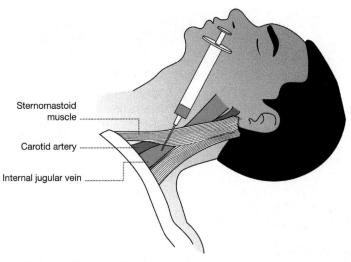

Figure 2.8 Anatomy of the internal jugular vein.

- ○ Turn head to opposite side of insertion site.
- ○ Stand at patient's head, with procedure trolley on right hand side if right handed.
- ○ Identify anatomy and locate carotid pulsation in relation to anticipated insertion site (see Figure 2.8 and 2.9).
- ○ Vein may be distended and can often be seen or balloted.
- ○ Confirm anatomy (see Figures 2.10 and 2.11) and position of vein using ultrasound (see Figure 2.12), if available.
- High approach (see Figure 2.13).
  - ○ Medial border of sternal head of sternocleidomastoid muscle, just lateral to carotid artery.

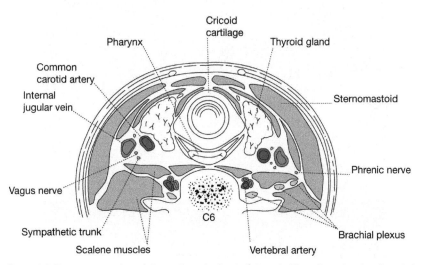

Figure 2.9 Transverse section of the neck at the level of the cricoid cartilage showing the relative anatomy of the internal jugular vein.

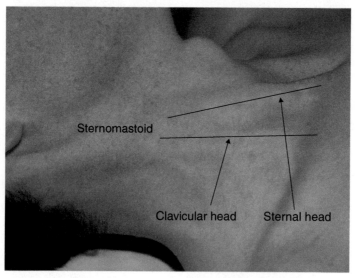

Figure 2.10 The triangle formed by the two heads of the sternocleidomastoid muscle.

- Middle approach (see Figure 2.13).
  - Insertion point at apex of triangle formed by the two heads of sternocleidomastoid muscle.
  - Advance needle along a line towards ipsilateral nipple.
- Low approach (see Figure 2.13):
  - Posterior border of sternal head of sternocleidomastoid muscle.
  - Higher risk of pneumothorax.
- Once blood is aspirated, proceed as per generic insertion technique.

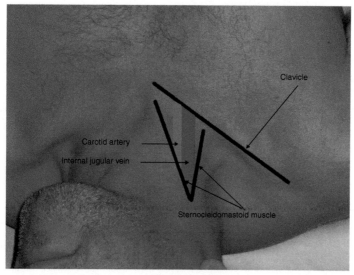

Figure 2.11 Surface anatomy of anterior neck with underlying structures illustrated.

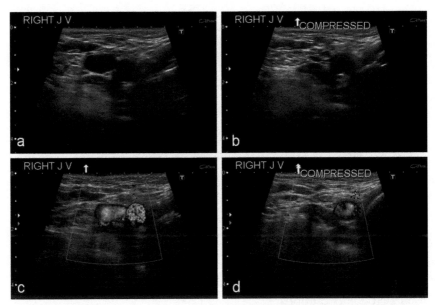

Figure 2.12 Images of the internal jugular vein anatomy. a. Internal jugular vein and carotid artery. b. External pressure using USS probe, compressing the internal jugular. c. Doppler demonstrating flow in both vessels. d. Doppler demonstrating no flow in internal jugular vein when compressed.

- Request a CXR after either a successful procedure or unsuccessful attempts (see Figure 2.14).
  - A pneumothorax may occur even, or especially, if line insertion is unsuccessful.
  - The operator must **personally** review the CXR.
    - Beware: pneumothorax may not be apparent on the first film. It may develop up to 36 hours later.
    - If patient is ventilated, tension pneumothorax may occur.

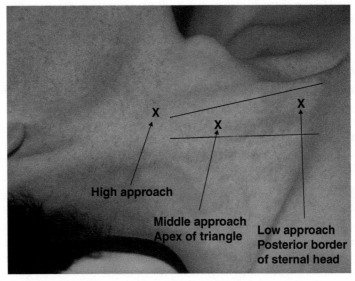

Figure 2.13 High, middle and low approaches to the internal jugular vein.

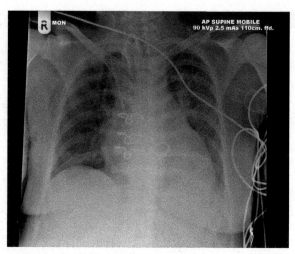

Figure 2.14 CXR of internal jugular CVC in correct position.

Important points/cautions

- The NICE recommended the use of ultrasound in every case, and not just in those that present difficulty (NICE, 2002).
- The internal jugular vein is usually relatively superficial while the Seldinger needles are relatively long. If the vein is not located within 2–4 cm of the needle breaking the skin, it is most likely that the vein has been missed.
  - The needle should be withdrawn slowly (whilst still aspirating gently in case the vein has been transfixed) and redirected.
- Advancing the Seldinger needle to the hilt greatly increases the risk of complications.

Tips and advice

- Head down positioning should help to distend the vein.
  - If already distended and anatomy easy to demonstrate, head-down positioning may not be required.
- Early use of ultrasound to identify anatomy is advised if difficulty anticipated:
  - e.g. in obese patients or those with prior use of neck for catheter placement.
- Always feel for arterial pulsation so the position of the carotid artery is identified.

References/further reading

National Institute of Clinical Excellence (2002) *Central venous catheters - ultrasound locating devices (TA49)*. http://guidance.nice.org.uk/TA49

Subclavian vein CVC insertion

Indications

- Useful site for longer term use.
  - Easy to secure the catheter to the chest wall, reducing movement at insertion site and therefore infection rate.

Contraindications

- Coagulopathy
- Anatomy of area means that it is difficult to apply pressure in the event of bleeding (either venous or arterial):
  - in comparison with the internal jugular or femoral approaches.
- Abnormal anatomy:
  - e.g. previous clavicular fracture.
- Severe lung disease:
  - in these patients the sequelae of a pneumothorax could be catastrophic.

Complications

- Pneumothorax:
  - higher incidence than with internal jugular vein cannulation.
- Misplacement
- Catheter may advance in a cephalad direction, up the internal jugular vein.
  - Will be seen on CXR and CVC will require removal and resiting.
- Arterial puncture:
  - incidence lower than with internal jugular approach, but potentially difficult to deal with.
  - arterial dilation can result in massive haemorrhage and haemothorax.
- Phrenic nerve trauma
- Recurrent laryngeal nerve trauma
- Thrombosis is probably more common than realized.

Equipment

- As for generic technique (see earlier sections).
- Rolled up towel or intravenous fluid bag (1 litre) to place under shoulders.
- Ultrasound can be used (difficult to visualize anatomy so may not help).

Sites

- Left or right subclavian veins.

Insertion technique

- **Many different techniques have been described of which only one is detailed below.**
- As for generic technique with additional points as below.
  - Position patient in Trendelenburg position, as tolerated.
  - Lift patient's shoulders and place a rolled up towel or litre bag of IV fluid between scapulae to extend the spine.
  - Identify the relevant anatomy (see Figures 2.15 and 2.16).
  - Insertion point:
    - 1 cm below clavicle, at junction of the medial third and middle third of the clavicle.
  - Advance needle aiming towards the back of the sternal notch.
  - Guide needle gently under the clavicle.
    - Some practitioners advocate locating the clavicle initially by hitting it with the needle and then 'walking' the needle under the inferior border whilst

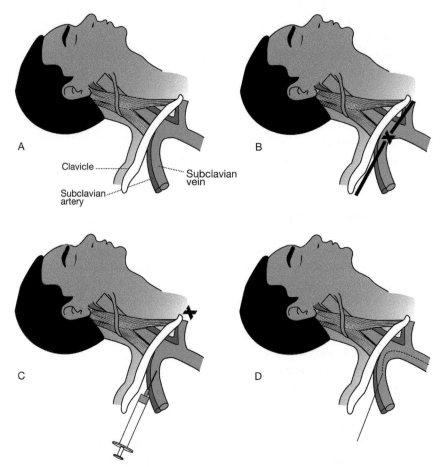

Figure 2.15 Anatomy of subclavian area.

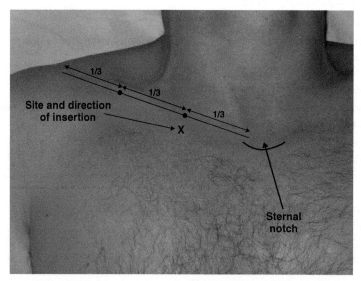

Figure 2.16 Surface anatomy for subclavian CVC insertion.

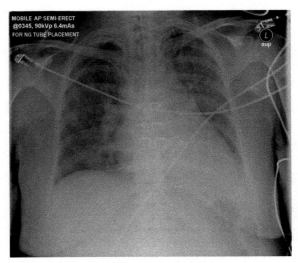

Figure 2.17 CXR with correctly positioned right subclavian CVC.

keeping the needle as horizontal as possible to avoid the dome of the pleura.
- ○ Once blood is aspirated continue as per generic insertion technique.
- ● Request a CXR (see Figure 2.17) after either a successful procedure or an unsuccessful attempt. This must be reviewed personally by the operator. Be aware that a pneumothorax may take time to develop and be visible.

Important points/cautions
- ● If arterial puncture occurs, withdraw needle and apply firm pressure both above and below clavicle.

Tips and advice
- ● If difficulty is encountered in locating the vein, ask an assistant to pull caudally on ipsilateral arm to move clavicle slightly.
- ● If a chest drain is in situ (e.g. following chest trauma) place CVC on **same** side as the drain, thereby avoiding the possibility of bilateral pneumothoraces/chest trauma.

Femoral vein CVC insertion

Indications
- ● As for generic CVC insertion.
- ● May be preferred site if coagulopathy exists.
  - ○ Direct pressure easily applied if complications on insertion (e.g. arterial puncture).
- ● Preferred site in:
  - ○ head and neck surgery (if CVC would be within operative field)
  - ○ with proven or possible raised ICP.
- ● Good for emergency access, even in hypovolaemic patients.
- ● Anatomy relatively constant.
- ● Good flow with large catheters (e.g. vascaths).
  - ○ More reliable as less kinking within vessels.

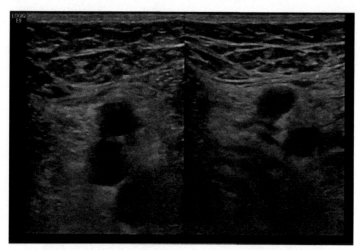

Figure 2.18 Variation in femoral vein and artery anatomy demonstrated with USS. USS Left common femoral vein beneath (deep to) femoral artery. Vein compresses showing no clot. Groin is to the left of the screen.

Contraindications
- As for generic CVC insertion
- Thrombosis in deep veins of leg

Complications
- As for generic CVC insertion

Equipment
- As for generic CVC insertion
- Ultrasound may be helpful in conjunction with anatomical landmarks (see Figures 2.18 and 2.19)

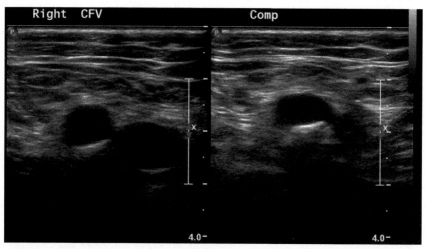

Figure 2.19 Variation in femoral vein and artery anatomy demonstrated with USS. USS Right common femoral vein. Vein on right of artery (demonstrating benefit of compressing even if not looking for clot, to confirm it is the vein, as the artery will not compress with gentle pressure).

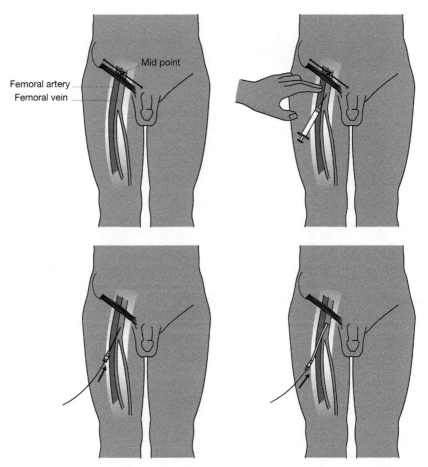

Femoral artery
Femoral vein
Mid point

Figure 2.20 Diagram demonstrating the anatomy of femoral triangle.

Sites

- Left or right femoral veins

Insertion technique

- As for generic insertion technique.
- Stand on patient's right if right-handed for cannulation of both left and right femoral veins (and vice versa for left handed operators).
- Identify anatomy (see Figures 2.20 and 2.21):
  - insertion point is 1–2 cm below inguinal ligament, 1–2 cm medial to femoral artery pulsation.
- Aim needle cephalad at 45-degree angle to skin.
- Continue as for generic insertion technique.

Important points/cautions

- Area is prone to local bacterial contamination.
- Transduced pressure may not correlate to true central venous pressure.

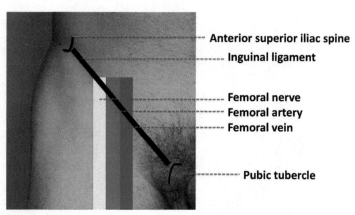

Figure 2.21 Surface anatomy for femoral vein cannulation with underlying structures illustrated.

Tips and advice

- If you are right handed stand on patient's right, regardless of side being cannulated.

External jugular vein cannulation

- This superficial vein lends itself to easy cannulation and is often visible overlying the sternomastoid, especially if the patient is in the head down position.
- It is not a 'blind' technique as the vein should be clearly visible.

Indications

- Cannulation in the emergency setting when peripheral access proves difficult.
- Can be chosen electively (beware contraindications – see below) as a site for central venous cannulation but long catheters are often difficult to pass.
- May be safer to cannulate in the presence of a coagulopathy.

Contraindications

- Should not be used as a site for long-term catheters due to infection risk.
- Coagulopathy;
  - However, this may be the preferred site in the presence of a coagulopathy, as direct pressure is easily applied.

Complications

- Localized bleeding and haematoma formation.
- Trauma to other structures in the neck:
  - Trachea, nerves, arterial puncture etc.
- Often, it proves difficult to pass a wire or catheter down the vein, due to either the constriction where the vein pierces the deep cervical fascia or a valve at the junction of the external jugular and subclavian veins.
- Thrombosis and thrombophlebitis:
  - This vein should really be regarded as a peripheral vein with regard to potential for catheter related infections.
- Pneumothorax (low risk).

Equipment

- CVC as per generic technique
- As an alternative, single lumen catheters, short and long

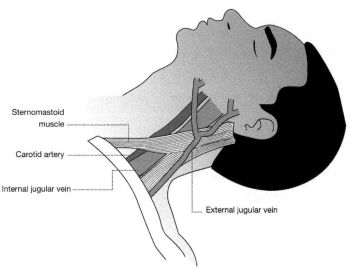

Figure 2.22 External jugular vein anatomy.

Sites

- Right or left external jugular vein

Insertion technique

- As for generic insertion technique.
- Place patient head down and head to one side, exposing the vein, as for insertion of an internal CVC.
- Identify anatomy (see Figures 2.22 and 2.23).
- Ensure vein is distended.
- Entry point should be around the mid-point of the sternocleidomastoid.

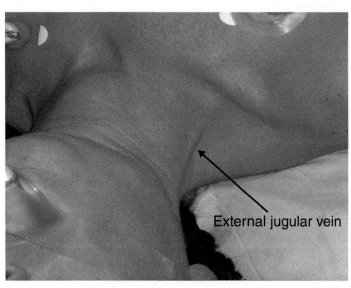

Figure 2.23 Surface anatomy of external jugular vein.

Tips and advice

- The right side is usually the most successful route.
- Encourage distension of the vein prior to needle insertion by placing the patient head down or applying pressure at the root of the neck. This will facilitate needle puncture.
- If difficulty is encountered passing the wire try gently rotating the wire on insertion or altering the position of the head.
- Ensure a CXR is performed following the procedure as the catheter does not reliably enter the subclavian vein following a central route.

Tunnelled central venous lines

- Tunnelled central venous lines are often inserted as a surgical procedure under general anaesthetic, however some are inserted under local anaesthesia with or without sedation.
- This technique is rarely employed by anaesthetists as it is usually only considered in patients who require long term venous access and who are at minimal risk of hospital acquired infection (i.e. lower risk for requiring removal of catheter in the event of acquiring a potentially blood-borne infection).
- Therefore we will not focus on the insertion of these lines, rather the removal of these lines as more often junior anaesthetic or intensive care staff may be required to remove these lines. It is important to understand how these lines are inserted in order to be able to remove them safely if required.

Indications

- Requirement for long term venous access.
  - Reduced incidence of catheter related infections as the site of insertion can be moved so as to be remote from potentially infected areas, e.g. a tracheostomy site.
  - Often used for long term cytotoxic drug regimens and parenteral nutrition delivery.
- Otherwise as for generic CVC.

Contraindications

- As for generic CVC.

Complications

- As for generic CVC.
- More prone to blockage if not cared for properly.

Equipment

- A catheter of tissue compatible material, such as silicone, with a Dacron cuff which is placed subcutaneously.

Sites

- As for generic CVC but most commonly subclavian.

Insertion technique

- There is a generic technique for inserting a tunnelled line (Hickman style with cuff).
- Full aseptic technique is **mandatory** as the line is intended to stay in situ for long periods.
- Decide on the site of skin entry with the patient.
  - Considerations include comfort, clothing and scarring.

- Inject local anaesthetic at the site where line will enter into the skin, the site of the wire insertion and the path between the two.
- Using a Seldinger technique insert the wire into the vein as for a subclavian line.
- Check position of the wire with image intensifier.
- Make a small incision at the insertion point of the wire and use blunt dissection to open a small space beneath wire entry site.
  - This is to accommodate the catheter as it turns to pass down into the vein.
- Make a small incision at the site where the catheter will enter the skin.
- Use blunt dissection to create a small pouch that will accommodate the cuff about 1–2 cm in from the skin surface.
- Measure the length from the entry site to the wire and to the approximate final position of the catheter, in the central vein at the right atrium.
- Cut the proximal catheter to the appropriate length.
- Attach the catheter to the supplied tunneller.
- Push the tunneller from the skin insertion site to the entry point of the wires.
- Pull the catheter until the cuff is snug in its subcutaneous pouch.
- Insert the introducer and dilator over the wire and into the vein.
- Remove the dilator ensuring no air is entrained into the introducer and thread the catheter (now removed from the tunneller) down through the introducer.
- The introducer will peel away (splitting in two) leaving the catheter beneath the skin.
  - Ensure it is seated comfortably and does not 'tent'.
- Check position with image intensifier.
  - The catheter should sit at the junction of the superior vena cava and right atrium.
- Ensure easy aspiration of blood through the catheter.
- Close the skin over the catheter.
- Close the skin entry site.
- Request a CXR to confirm correct catheter position.

Removal technique

- This should be conducted in as sterile a manner as possible and it is therefore considered as a minor surgical procedure.
- The subcutaneous cuff is designed to secure the catheter by promoting local tissue adherence and is therefore often difficult to remove.
- Examine the patient and ensure that the cuff position can be identified.
  - Sometimes a gentle tug on the line will indicate where it is tethered as some practitioners place the cuff some distance from the skin to reduce the likelihood of the line coming out – it may be difficult to feel the cuff and even more difficult to remove.
- Prepare equipment:
  - sterile gown, gloves and drapes
  - chlorhexidine or iodine based skin preparation solution
  - minor surgical pack containing scalpel, artery forceps, skin suture, gauze and dressings
  - local anaesthetic for skin infiltration with appropriate needle and syringe.

- Prepare patient as required:
  - informed consent
  - sedation
  - clean and drape.
- Infiltrate skin with local anaesthetic.
- Make 1–2 cm incision over palpable subcutaneous catheter cuff and dissect around cuff using blunt dissection.
- Once cuff is free of surrounding tissue clamp the distal end of the catheter (the part that goes from the cuff into the vein i.e. furthest from the operator) with artery forceps so as not to 'lose' the distal end of the catheter into the patient.
- Transect the catheter above the cuff.
- Gently withdraw the distal part of the catheter until it is out of both the vein and the patient.
- Then withdraw the whole catheter from the patient.
  - If the cuff is close to the skin and mobilized then the whole catheter can be easily withdrawn.
  - If the cuff is far removed from the skin entry site, then at this stage (*and not before*) it might be necessary to transect the distal catheter (no longer in the patient) so that both ends of the catheter can be removed without having to pull the cuff through a long subcutaneous tunnel.
- Never lose control of the distal catheter (the part in the vein).
- Apply pressure to the removal site if bleeding occurs.
- Suture skin incision.
- Apply dressing.
- Document procedure in notes.

Important points/cautions

- Caution in presence of coagulopathy.

Tips and advice

- Always identify the location of the cuff before starting.
- It should be possible to withdraw the catheter with minimal force and the need for excessive force can be reduced with further blunt dissection if required.
- Avoid applying excessive force when withdrawing the catheter as this increases the risk of catheter fracture.
- Never pull the catheter – they can, and do, break.

Peripheral sites for central venous access: peripherally inserted central catheter (PICC) lines

Indications

- As for all CVCs
- Difficulty in siting CVC via alternative routes
- To avoid risk of pneumothorax
- In presence of coagulopathy:
  - Haemorrhage caused by the cannula can be controlled by local pressure.

Contraindications

- Absolute:
  - vein thrombosed and occluded.

- Relative:
  - patient refusal
  - local sepsis or injury e.g. burns
  - coagulopathy
  - obesity (may be difficult)
  - difficult or very small peripheral veins.

Complications
- Common:
  - failure to cannulate vein
  - difficulty passing catheter past the axilla
  - arterial puncture
  - infection
  - venous thrombosis.
- Rare
  - air embolism
  - neurapraxia (median nerve).

Equipment
- 50–60 cm, 2–5F, single or double lumen Peripherally Inserted Central Catheter (PICC)
- Ametop anaesthetic cream or local anaesthetic for subcutaneous infiltration
- Tape measure
- Tourniquet
- Sterile pack
- Antiseptic solution
- Saline or heparinized saline for flushing lines
- Consider 14-gauge cannula as spare introducer
- Sterile semi-permeable adhesive dressing

Sites
- Basilic vein (medial antecubital fossa)
- Cephalic vein (lateral antecubital fossa)
- Median cubital vein

Insertion technique
- Explain the procedure and gain patient's consent.
- Ideally, an assistant should be available.
- Prepare the patient:
  - position patient appropriately (supine if possible).
  - Identify the anatomy and ensure suitable vein (see Figure 2.24).
  - Estimate the required length of catheter to be inserted. There are a number of methods to achieve this. One is to extend the patient's arm 90 degrees to their body and measure the distance from the insertion site to the head of humerus and across to the sternoclavicular junction.
- Prepare the equipment:
  - Think through the steps involved and ensure all equipment required is available and to hand.

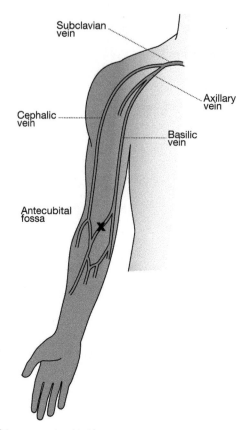

Figure 2.24 Veins of the arm – antecubital fossa.

- Full aseptic technique – **important**!
  - Even with a peripheral insertion site, sterility is very important as these lines are generally intended for longer-term use.
- Open the equipment and prepare.
  - Consider the length of catheter to be inserted. Generally a 50 cm line is inserted but the length may need to be reduced (e.g. in paediatric patients) to reflect the estimated distance from insertion site to superior vena cava.
- Clean the skin with antiseptic.
- Prepare sterile field with drape.
  - Ideally a large transparent drape with precut fenestration.
- Infiltrate skin with local anaesthetic.
  - Massage area to avoid distortion of anatomy.
- Cannulate the vein with the introducer needle.
- Remove needle.
- Insert catheter into the introducer cannula and advance to a depth of about 40–50 cm (depending on estimated length required).
- Withdraw introducer cannula ensuring catheter remains in situ (the cannula usually peels along its sides for removal).
- Remove stiffening wire if present.

- Connect proximal end of catheter appropriately (depending on manufacturer of specific PICC line in use).
- Stitch hub in place (if appropriate).
- Cover with sterile transparent semi-permeable dressing.
- Request a CXR to ensure correct placement.
- Document procedure in patients notes.

Important points/cautions

- The catheter may not always reach an intrathoracic vein and may therefore be unreliable for measuring central venous pressure.
- The catheter rarely passes cephalad into the internal jugular vein.
  - Check correct positioning on the CXR.

Tips and advice

- Insertion on the medial aspect of the ante-cubital fossa provides a less tortuous route for the catheter. The cephalic vein (lateral side) often has a valve that prevents cannulation, and entry into the thorax through the clavipectoral fascia is at a more acute angle.
- The catheter is occasionally difficult to pass past the axilla.
  - Try abducting the arm and advancing again.
  - Alternatively flush catheter with saline while advancing.

'Special' lines

Pulmonary artery catheter

- There is ongoing debate regarding the place of pulmonary artery catheters (PACs) in the care of critically ill patients. The risks associated with their use (e.g. pulmonary artery rupture) are small but do exist; however, significant information can be gained about a patient's physiology through their use.
- PACs were widely used for many years, but recently their use has declined. This is probably as a result of evidence arising that suggests PAC use is not associated with an improved outcome in an intensive care setting (Harvey et al. 2005), together with the development and more widespread use of less invasive techniques for gathering similar haemodynamic information (e.g. oesophageal Doppler, PICCO and LIDCO systems), which have lower risk of patient morbidity.

Indications

- There are no absolute indications for insertion of a PAC as the benefits and risks of insertion must be weighed up on an individual basis.
- Essentially a PAC can be considered for specific disease states where central venous pressure no longer correlates with filling pressures of both right and left atria as in normal individuals. Although not exhaustive, examples include:
  - pulmonary hypertension
  - left ventricular failure with pulmonary oedema
  - interstitial pulmonary oedema
  - chronic pulmonary disease
  - valvular heart disease.
- In these conditions the PAC will be able to achieve:
  - measurement of pulmonary artery (PA) pressures
  - measurement of pulmonary artery occlusion pressure (PAoP).
    - this reflects the left atrial pressure and can be used as an index of left ventricular function
  - measurement of cardiac output:
    - using thermodilution
  - sampling:
    - blood aspirated from the pulmonary artery will be true mixed-venous blood
  - measurement of many other haemodynamic parameters that can be derived from the directly measured values above, such as the pulmonary vascular resistance, and oxygen delivery and uptake
  - utility for direction of management based on oxygen delivery.

Contraindications

Relative:

- coagulopathy or thrombocytopenia, due to large bore introducer used
- pacemaker in situ
- prosthetic heart valves
- severe mitral regurgitation
- pulmonary hypertension
- septal defects
- cardiac arrhythmias.

Complications

- As for generic CVC insertion
- Air entrainment due to large bore introducer
- Cardiac dysrhythmias
- Pulmonary artery rupture (in up to 0.2% of patients):
  - Reduce risk by minimizing balloon inflation in the PA and monitoring the PA trace continuously in order to detect spontaneous wedging as a result of unintended catheter migration.
- Pulmonary infarction:
  - Again, as a result of spontaneous PA wedging
- Knotting/coiling of catheter:
  - Avoid by limiting the length of catheter inserted without a change in the pressure waveform
- Balloon rupture
- Valve damage
- Sepsis (including endocarditis)

Equipment

- As for generic CVC insertion with the addition of:
  - pulmonary artery catheter introducer set
  - pulmonary artery catheter
  - monitoring to display pressure waveforms during insertion
  - cardiac output computer (usually contained within standard monitors on ICU with additional modules)
  - injectate giving set and ice cold water.

Sites

- Any site, as for any CVC insertion, may be used but the right internal jugular and left subclavian veins allow best use of the natural curvature of the catheter.

Insertion technique

Introducer sheath

- Select access site.
- Obtain patient consent and use aseptic technique as per generic CVC insertion.
- Arrange the PAC introducer for use (note: the dilator is often pre-loaded into the introducer cannula and will need to be removed if flushed prior to insertion).
- Flush the PAC introducer.
- Locate vein with needle or cannula and insert guidewire.
- Remove needle/cannula leaving the guidewire in place.
- Make small incision in skin at entry point of wire to aid insertion.
- The dilator and introducer catheter are inserted as one and this is often difficult. The combination is large bore, stiff and long so care must be taken.
  - Often the skin must be held taut, and a twisting motion may aid insertion.
- The dilator rarely, if ever, needs to be inserted fully and the introducer should slide over the dilator into the vein.
- Remove dilator.
- Aspirate and flush catheter.

Pulmonary Artery Catheter

- Additional preparation of the PAC:
  - Test the integrity of the PAC balloon by inflating with **air, not saline.**
  - Flush the proximal and distal lumen with saline, attaching three-way taps.
  - Attach the distal lumen to the pressure transducer tubing, ensuring no bubbles enter the system.
  - Calibrate and zero the transducer, setting an appropriate scale (0-60 mmHg is usual).
- Lay the PAC on the drapes to ensure ease of insertion.
- With balloon **deflated** insert the catheter into the introducer and advance to 20 cm to ensure the balloon is beyond the end of the introducer.
- Inflate the balloon.
- Advance the catheter whilst watching the pressure waveform (see Figure 2.25) and ECG trace. A change in pattern will be seen on passing from SVC to atria, ventricle and pulmonary artery.
- If the catheter has been advanced further than 10 cm without a change in waveform the catheter is probably coiling.
  - Deflate the balloon, withdraw and reattempt insertion.
- The pulmonary artery is usually 40-50 cm from the internal jugular and a characteristic waveform will be seen.
- On advancing further, the pulmonary arterial trace disappears, leaving a flatter trace known as the wedge.
- Deflate the balloon and ensure the pulmonary trace reappears (this indicates there is flow around the catheter).
- Note the depth of catheter insertion, secure the catheter and apply sterile dressings.
- Request a CXR to ensure correct placement.

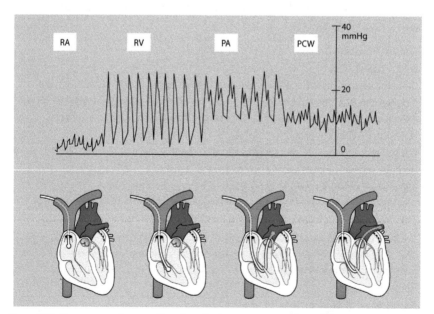

Figure 2.25 Pressure waveforms on insertion of pulmonary artery catheter. RA, right atrial trace; RV, right ventricular trace; PA, pulmonary artery trace; PCW, wedge trace (variation with respiration).

Tips and advice

- The ECG must be observed throughout.
- Treat dysrhythmias by withdrawing catheter in the first instance.
  - ○ Ensure defibrillator is to hand and consider use of lidocaine before re-attempting insertion.
- **Always** deflate balloon before withdrawing catheter to avoid valve damage.
- Ensure balloon is deflated when not taking measurements.
- Only ever inflate the balloon with air, never water/saline.
- The pressure waveform must be displayed constantly.
  - ○ A flat trace is due to wedging unless proved otherwise.
    - ■ Other causes include kinking (often at point of insertion through skin) or internal occlusion.

References/further reading

Harvey S et al. (2005). Assessment of the clinical effectiveness of pulmonary artery catheters in management of patients in intensive care (PAC-Man): a randomized controlled trial. *The Lancet* 366 p. 472–477

Sandham JD, Hull RD, Brant RF et al. (2003). A randomized, controlled trial of the use of pulmonary-artery catheters in high-risk surgical patients. *New England Journal of Medicine*, 348 p. 5–14.

Polanczyk CA, Rohde LE, Goldman L, et al. (2001). Right heart catheterization and cardiac complications in patients undergoing noncardiac surgery: an observational study. *JAMA*, 286 p. 309–314.

Dalen JE, Bone RC (1996). Is it time to pull the pulmonary artery catheter? *JAMA*, 276 p. 916–8

Connors AF (2002). Equipoise, power, and the pulmonary artery catheter. *Intensive Care Medicine*, 28 p. 225–6.

Connors AF Jr, Speroff T, Dawson NV, et al. (1996). The effectiveness of right heart catheterization in the initial care of critically ill patients. *JAMA*, 276 p. 889–897.

Bernard GR, Sopko G, Cerra F, et al. (2000). Pulmonary artery catheterization and clinical outcomes: National Heart, Lung, and Blood Institute and Food and Drug Administration Workshop Report: consensus statement. *JAMA*, 283 p. 2568–72.

Greenberg SB, Murphy GS, Vender JS (2009). Current use of the pulmonary artery catheter. *Current Opinion Critical Care*, 15 p. 249–53.

Intraosseous needle insertion

Indications

- 'Vascular access' in life threatening situations in children.
- Following three failed attempts at intravenous access (or greater than 90 seconds) in an acutely unwell child.
- Intravenous fluids, blood products and medication may be given via this route.
- Use in adults is being promoted (especially in battlefield resuscitation) but the technique is not widely used at present.

Contraindications

- Proximal limb fracture:
  - ○ May develop compartment syndrome.
- Infected skin or wounds overlying insertion point
- Bone structure abnormalities:
  - ○ Osteogenesis imperfecta/osteoporosis.

Complications

- Extravasation:
  - True extravasation due to misplacement of the needle is relatively uncommon and localized swelling may be seen even with correct placement due to lymphatic and perforator drainage from the bone. If in any doubt, stop infusion, aspirate from needle and confirm aspiration of marrow still possible.
- Embolisation:
  - Of fat or bone marrow, risk less than 1%.
- Infection:
  - Osteomyelitis
- Compartment syndrome
- Fracture
- Skin necrosis

Equipment

- Sterile pack, to maintain aseptic technique.
- Skin disinfectant.
- Local anaesthetic (if required).
- Appropriately sized intraosseous needle.
  - Most commonly a trocar needle with an end hole and two side holes for manual insertion, although there are also other styles available.
  - Neonate-6 months: 18G.
  - 6 months-18 months: 16G.
  - >18 months: 14G.
- 50 ml syringe.
- An electric drill to aid insertion is also now available but not currently widely used.

Sites

- Under 6 years of age (EPLS 2006):
  - anteromedial surface of the tibia 2–3 cm below the tibial tuberosity.
    - These sites are chosen in order to avoid the growth plates of the long bones (see Figure 2.26).
- Over 6 years of age (EPLS 2006):
  - medial aspect of the tibia, 3 cm above the medial malleolus
  - lateral aspect of the femur, 3 cm above the lateral condyle.
    - These sites are chosen in order to avoid the growth plates of the long bones.
- Adult (ALS 2006):
  - Proximal tibia (2 cm below the tibial tuberosity on the anteromedial side)
  - Distal tibia (2 cm proximal to the medial malleolus).

Insertion technique

- Ensure correct equipment is available and prepared.
- Identify landmarks and chose entry site.
- Immobilize limb with either non-dominant hand or with assistance.
  - Do not place hand under the limb - risk of needle injury.

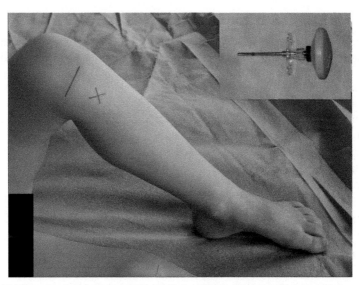

Figure 2.26 Insertion sites for intraosseous needle in children under age of 6 years, with intraosseous needle (inset). The line indicates the level of the tibial tuberosity; X indicates the insertion point 2–3 cm below on the anteromedial surface of the tibia.

- Infiltrate with local anaesthetic down to periosteum.
- Insert needle at 90 degrees (perpendicular) to skin.
- Advance the needle with a rotating/drilling action until a give is felt as the cortex of the bone is penetrated.
- Remove the trocar.
- Aspirate to confirm correct placement.
  - It should be possible to aspirate bone marrow.
  - If appropriate, remember to take samples for relevant laboratory analyses e.g. full blood count, urea and electrolytes, group and save or crossmatch.
- Attach a three-way tap and a primed fluid giving set.
- Either infuse under gentle pressure or by using a 50 ml syringe attached to the three-way tap.
- Secure the needle in position using tape.

Important points/cautions

- If doubt as to correct placement then remove and reinsert, possibly in the contralateral limb.

Tips and advice

- This is probably an underused technique for many anaesthetists and should perhaps be considered earlier than traditionally done so in the resuscitation of children.

References/further reading

European Resuscitation Council (2006). Vascular Access. *European Paediatric Life Support.* p. 33–4. Resuscitation Council (UK), London.
UK Resuscitation Council (2006) *Advanced Life Support. 5th Edition.*

Lines for haemofiltration/dialysis

- The most common method of management of the consequences of acute renal failure (in the acute setting) is now continuous renal replacement therapy (CRRT). Either continuous venovenous haemofiltration (CVVH) or continuous venovenous haemodialysis (CVVHD), or a combination of both (continuous venovenous haemodiafiltration (CVVHDF) may be undertaken. Previous methods such as intermittent haemodialysis (IHD) and arteriovenous haemofiltration have largely been replaced and will not be discussed further.
- Vocabulary:
  - C is continuous
  - VV is venovenous (pump)
  - A-V is arteriovenous (not currently used)
  - HD is haemodialysis
  - HF haemofiltration
  - HDF haemodiafiltration
  - UF ultrafiltration

Indications

Main:
- uraemia
- fluid overload/pulmonary oedema
- hyperkalaemia.

Relative:
- cooling patients.

Controversial:
- acidosis.

Contraindications

- As for CVC insertion.
- Large bore catheters are used and therefore greater risk is entailed if coagulopathy exists.

Complications

- As for CVC insertion.
- Additionally:
  - risk of air embolism (due to need for mechanical pump)
  - risk of disconnection and rapid exsanguination
  - risk of bleeding (especially if pump circuit anticoagulated; although this is not necessary, it might prolong filter life).
- Hypotensive and hypoxic episodes on initiation of haemofiltration.

Equipment

- As for CVC insertion (minus CVC line)
- CVVHD circuit using a simple blood pump, with pumps for dialysate control
- A double lumen venous catheter:
  - 15 cm for right internal jugular and right subclavian lines
  - 20 cm for left internal jugular, left subclavian or femoral (right and left) lines
  - an additional, smaller gauge, lumen (optional).

Sites

- Femoral vein:
  - often preferred as lower risk of kinking of line
  - in presence of coagulopathy, pressure is more easily applied if required.
- Internal jugular vein:
  - anatomically more challenging to insert and prone to kinking, particularly from the left.
- Subclavian vein:
  - provides good access but can kink under the clavicle and best avoided in presence of coagulopathy.

Insertion technique

- As for generic CVC insertion.
- Prepare by flushing all lumens with saline and clamping them off.
- Locate vein using preferred method and insert using the Seldinger technique (see earlier section).
- Ensure blood is freely aspirated from all lumens (free flow of blood will be required in order for optimum pump function).
- Suture in position, noting the depth of insertion, and cover with sterile dressing.
- Request a CXR if placed in internal jugular or subclavian veins.

Important points/cautions

- The catheter is large bore.
  - Significant pressure may be required during insertion. Reduce this by ensuring skin incision at site of Seldinger wire and holding the skin taut on insertion.
  - Consequently the dilator is long, so use caution, especially if inserting in internal jugular or subclavian veins.

Tips and advice

- Ensure free flow of blood from both lumens at time of placement.
  The haemofiltration pump will be unable to run without good access pressures (i.e. flow) and will only have to be replaced if inadequate. It is worth ensuring good position at time of insertion.
- Blood flow rates in adults:
  - approx. 150 ml/min
  - dialysate approx. 2 L/hr
- Remember anticoagulation:
  - heparin or prostacyclin.
- One author always closes the skin around the entry site in order to reduce movement and bleeding.
- Essentially these are the methods by which these devices function:
  - Hydrostatic pressure pushes fluid and small molecules across the filter (convection). Alternatively, an osmotic gradient pulls fluid and small molecules across the membrane, in dialysis (diffusion). These mechanisms can be combined.
  - Filtration methods require infusion of fluid into the circulation proximal to the filter, which is then filtered back out with associated molecules. Hence the clearance equates to the amount filtered. At 2 L/hr this equates to 33 ml/min. In 24 hours, 48 litres of fluid will have been infused into the blood at the filter.

○ Dialysis requires the dialysate to be on the other side of the membrane from the blood, and the dialysate does not enter the blood stream. At 150 ml/min blood flow and 2 L/min dialysate flow, a clearance of 25–30 ml/min is often achieved. During a 24 hour period no dialysate is infused into the blood.

Dialysis

● The principles of dialysis in its various modes are too broad to be covered here. A brief overview will suffice.

Indications
Absolute:

● to treat fluid overload e.g. in renal failure
● to treat hyperkalaemia
● to remove urea and creatinine.
  ○ A urea concentration of 30mmol/l is often used as a value at which dialysis should be considered.

Relative:

● Correcting acid-base abnormalities:
  ○ it is effective in correcting renal acidosis that is due to retained fixed acids which is usually mild and takes time to accumulate.
  ○ it will not address the other causes of acidosis such as lactic acidosis but is nonetheless enjoying a renaissance for treating acidosis.
● Removing poisons with polar molecules, low protein binding and small volume of distribution.
● As an extracorporeal circuit to cool patients.

General principles

● Fluid and small molecules can move across semi-permeable membranes.
● The pressures involved are either hydrostatic or osmolar.
● Fluid moving will have solute drag, and thus pulls molecules with it. This is convection.
● Dialysis is the movement of molecules down concentration gradients. There is inevitably some associated fluid movement.

Concepts (see Figure 2.27)

● Dialysis can be intermittent or continuous. The former is often high flow and intensive (performed at renal units); the latter has lower flow and lower clearance but is done continuously.
● The driving force pushing the blood through the filter alongside the membrane can be that from arteriovenous flow or can be generated by an endogenous pump. The latter is more common now.
  ○ Flow is in the order of 150 ml/min in most continuous systems.
● Ultrafiltration:
  ○ Uses hydrostatic pressure to push fluid and electrolytes through the membrane and away.
    ■ Used to rapidly remove fluid.
● Haemofiltration
  ○ Filters fluid and hence other molecules, such as urea and creatinine, from the blood. As flow rates in the order of 2 L/hr are achieved the fluid is replaced by

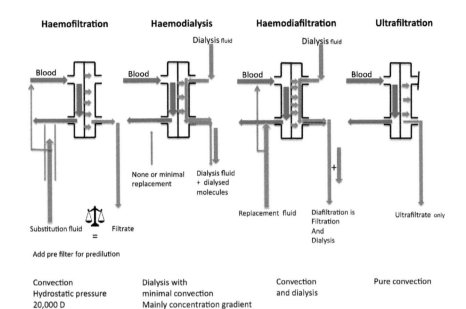

Figure 2.27 Different methods of dialysis and filtration.

a dialysate fluid. This is given back into the circuit so there is no reduction in intravascular volume, unless this is desired.

- ○ 2 L/hr filtration is equivalent to about 30 ml/min clearance.
- Haemodialysis:
  - ○ Haemodialysis dialysate is passed as a counter-current on the other side of the dialysis membrane from the blood. The concentration gradients drive molecular movement with some passive fluid shift.
  - ○ Although efficient at removing molecules such as urea, there is minimal fluid loss and no need for replacement.
  - ○ 2 L/hr dialysate flow will produce clearance in the order of 30 ml/min; this is marginally less than with haemofiltration and is dependent on membrane function. Dialysis against a standard solution protects the patient against excessive electrolyte loss.
- Haemodiafiltration:
  - ○ The combination of filtration and dialysis. There is a requirement for both fluid replacement of filtration fluid and the use of dialysis fluid. Much more dialysate fluid is therefore required, with some increase in clearance. This increase has not been shown to be beneficial.
  - ○ Hypophosphataemia may be an issue.

References/further reading

Bellomo R (2000). Continuous haemofiltration in the intensive care unit. *Critical Care* 4 p. 339–45.

Arterial line insertion

Indications
- Continuous blood pressure monitoring
- Repeated sampling

Contraindications
- Absolute:
  - none.
- Relative:
  - local sepsis
  - coagulopathy
  - no collateral circulation detected on Allen's test.

Complications
- Haematoma:
  - Limit with firm pressure for 3 minutes
- Dissection
- Thrombosis
- Aneurysm formation
- Inadvertent drug injection:
  - Label the line clearly
- Line sepsis
- Ischaemia of the hand

Equipment
- 20G or 22G Abbocath (32 mm or 51 mm)
- 20G BD Insyte (30 mm or 48 mm)
- 20G Vygon Leader Cath (Seldinger technique)

Sites
- Choose the site where a pulse can easily be felt, that is accessible and where the cannula can be secured easily.
- Radial artery:
  - Preferred site as easily accessible, superficial and collateral circulation usually exists (assess with Allen's test if doubt).
- Brachial artery
- Femoral artery
- Dorsalis pedis artery
- Posterior tibial artery

Insertion technique for radial artery
- Perform Allen's Test.
  - It is important that collateral arterial flow is adequate. Compress radial artery at wrist and look for blanching of the hand. Blanching is a contraindication to using that vessel for cannulation.
- Use aseptic technique.
- Hyperextend wrist (see Figure 2.28). A 500 ml bag of fluid works well.
- Clean skin thoroughly (see section on aseptic technique).

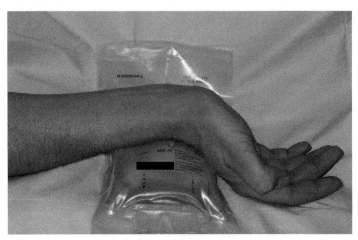

Figure 2.28 Positioning of wrist for insertion of arterial line.

- Infiltrate local anaesthetic over point of insertion and massage to avoid distorting anatomy.
- Hold cannula like a pencil and insert through skin at a 30-degree angle to skin surface.
- Advance cannula until flashback seen and either:
  - advance cannula as if cannulating a vein, or:
  - advance cannula through the other side of the vessel. Withdraw the needle partially or completely and attach a 2 ml syringe to the cannula. Withdraw the cannula slowly until blood pours freely from it and advance cannula into the artery (whilst removing needle if still in cannula).
- Connect pressurized line and flush with saline.
- Secure cannula, apply sterile dressing and connect transducer.

Seldinger technique

- Steps 1–6 as above, using 20G introducer needle.
- Advance needle until artery located (pulsatile blood).
- Insert wire through needle.
- Remove needle over wire.
- Advance cannula over wire into artery. Maintain contact with wire throughout.
- Remove wire and connect line and secure as above.

Tips and advice

- Choosing a site in the forearm proximal to the wrist reduces the incidence of line occlusion due to wrist flexion.
- A wire can be inserted into a cannula if it is difficult to advance the cannula over the needle.
- If difficulty advancing cannula is encountered despite it being easy to aspirate try rotating cannula whilst advancing.

Rapid infusion devices

- These allow rapid infusion of warmed fluids.
- Flow performance will be dictated by the narrowest section of the system:
  - usually the cannula in the vessel, so large cannulae will produce better performance
  - flow rates are usually up to about 500 ml/min but some larger devices can achieve 1400 ml/min.
- It is important to know the capabilities and limitations of each individual device.

Indications

- Any situation where there is a requirement for rapid large volume infusion. This includes blood and some blood products, colloids and crystalloids. (Note: it is not appropriate for platelets, cryoprecipitate or granulocytes.)
- Rapid infusion of warmed fluids:
  - massive haemorrhage, anticipated or unanticipated
  - prevention of hypothermia, which may contribute to coagulopathy.
- Rewarming a cold patient – an adjunct.

Contraindications

- None, although it is important to ensure that the free-flowing cannula has been sited correctly due to the risk of extravasation.

Complications

- Extravasation
- The high infusion rate is a potential cause of fluid overload that can occur easily if patient is not properly monitored.
- Air embolus:
  - Potentially catastrophic due to speed of infusion.
  - As with any fluid administration there is inevitably the potential for air to enter the system, especially when new bags are being connected. Meticulous air exclusion is important but there should also be air detection systems in place on the device with both an automatic shut off and an alarm.

Equipment

- Rapid transfusion device:
  - Pressurized chambers, commonly up to 300 mmHg
  - Ability to warm fluids rapidly
  - Air detection device
  - Air elimination mechanism
  - Flow rate dependent on calibre and length of tubing and cannula

Sites

- Any site appropriate for a large bore cannula in a vein.

Insertion technique

- See previous sections.

Important points/cautions

- Always ensure you are familiar with the individual device in use and know how it works. In particular, be aware of how the air detection and prevention device functions and also how the heating system operates, so that it is set appropriately.

As with any equipment that is used intermittently, it must be properly maintained and serviced.

- Most devices use custom equipment sets and this may be important for proper functionality.
- This is a pressurized system, and the operating pressures are often around 300 mmHg. This has implications for leakage, flow performance and potential air entrainment.
- Ensure the equipment set used for delivery is fully primed prior to connection to the patient to avoid air embolisation.
- Infection control issues mandate meticulous cleanliness of the machine and careful use of the disposable circuits.

Transducers

Indications

- In the context of anaesthesia a transducer will convert a pressure waveform into an electrical signal.
- Pressure waveforms transduced:
  - Central venous pressure
  - Arterial pressure
  - ICP
  - Pulmonary arterial and pulmonary artery occlusion pressures.

Contraindications

- None

Complications

- Potential for inaccurate readings due to incorrect set-up with consequent incorrect management decisions.

Equipment

- Several different systems exist but the principles remain the same.
- Intravenous/Intra-arterial/Intracranial cannula
- Pressure transducer system:
  - Provides a continuous column of fluid between cannula and transducer
  - 500 ml bag 0.9% saline
  - 'Pressure bag' to pressurize saline bag to 300 mmHg
- Electrical monitor to provide a digital value or waveform

Sites

- Intravenous
- Intra-arterial
- Intracranial

Insertion technique

- How to calibrate to zero:
  - place the transducer at the level of the pressure to be measured (i.e. at the level of the atria if measuring central venous pressure)
  - open the system to the air (i.e. 'off to patient')
  - press the 'zero' function button on the monitor.

Important points/cautions

- Ensure that no air is present in the system.
  - Minimizes damping.
  - Reduces risk of air emboli.
- Maintain pressure within system.
  - Maintains patency of the line.
- Ensure system calibrated correctly.
  - 'Zero' regularly as systems can 'drift' dramatically during use.
- Watch for damping of the trace.
  - This may lead to inaccurate readings.
  - Usually resolved by flushing the line.

Chapter 3
Monitoring

'Routine' anaesthetic monitoring

> **Box 3.1 Monitoring Devices**
>
> **Recommendations for standards of monitoring during anaesthesia and recovery. (AAGBI 2007)**
>
> The following monitoring devices are essential to the safe conduct of anaesthesia. If it is necessary to continue anaesthesia without a particular device, the anaesthetist must clearly record the reasons for this in the anaesthetic record.
>
> ### A Induction and Maintenance of Anaesthesia
> 1 Pulse oximeter
> 2 Non-invasive blood pressure monitor
> 3 Electrocardiograph
> 4 Airway gases: oxygen, carbon dioxide and vapour
> 5 Airway pressure
>   The following must also be available:
> - a nerve stimulator whenever a muscle relaxant is used
> - a means of measuring the patient's temperature.
>
>   During induction of anaesthesia in children and in uncooperative adults it may not be possible to attach all monitoring before induction. In these circumstances monitoring must be attached as soon as possible and the reasons for delay recorded in the patient's notes.
>
> ### B Recovery from Anaesthesia
> A high standard of monitoring should be maintained until the patient is fully recovered from anaesthesia. Clinical observations must be supplemented by the following monitoring devices.
> 1 Pulse oximeter
> 2 Non-invasive blood pressure monitor
>   The following must also be immediately available:
> - electrocardiograph
> - nerve stimulator
> - means of measuring temperature
> - capnograph.
>
>   If the recovery area is not immediately adjacent to the operating theatre, or if the patient's general condition is poor, adequate mobile monitoring of the above parameters will be needed during transfer. The anaesthetist is responsible for ensuring that this transfer is accomplished safely.
>
> Reproduced with the kind permission of the Association of Anaesthetists of Great Britain and Ireland.

References/further reading

Association of Anaesthetists of Great Britain and Northern Ireland (2007). *Recommendations for Standards of Monitoring during Anaesthesia and Recovery*, 4th Edition. Published by The Association of Anaesthetists of Great Britain and Ireland, London.

12-lead ECG

- Electrocardiographs (ECG) are useful diagnostic devices. Discussion of their interpretation would require an entire book in its own right, so this section will concentrate on basic principles and how to record an ECG.
- There are two types of recording: bipolar and unipolar.
  - Bipolar recording measures the electrical potential between any two points. The standard leads, I, II and III, are positioned between the right and left arm, right arm and left leg and left arm and right leg respectively.
  - Unipolar leads use an electrode against an effective zero potential. They run between a central point V and the left arm, right arm and left leg (aVL, aVR and aVF, respectively). The unipolar precordial leads are denoted by V1-6.
- To record a 12-lead ECG one needs electrodes on all 4 limbs, and the precordial leads. The leads need to be in the appropriate positions and are usually labelled.
- The ECG machine will be programmed to then measure and record between the relevant electrodes.

Technique

- Prepare patient:
  - shave and clean appropriate areas for electrode placement
  - this improves contact between patient and electrode.
- Prepare equipment:
  - turn on machine
  - input patient data
  - check calibration.
    - Paper markings: horizontal lines show the amplitude and are 1 mm apart. By convention, 1 cm equates to 1 millivolt.
    - Vertical lines indicate time intervals: each small square represents 0.04 seconds at a paper speed of 25 mm/sec.
- Connect the leads to the appropriate electrodes.
  - Usually indicated on the leads to aid correct placement.
- Ask the patient to sit still, and avoid moving and speaking.
- Start the analysis.
  - The ECG machine will produce the standard, familiar 12 lead ECG with rhythm strip along the bottom of the page.

Tips and advice

- Where to place the chest leads (see Figure 3.1):
  - V1: Right sternal edge, 4th intercostal space
  - V2: Left sternal edge, 4th intercostal space
  - V3: Half-way between V2 and V4
  - V4: 5th intercostal space, mid clavicular line (apex beat)
  - V5: Level with V4, left anterior axillary line
  - V6: Level with V4, left mid axillary line.
- If poor recording obtained:
  - check the electrodes to ensure good contact with the patient's skin
  - artefact often seen with patient movement so repeat ensuring patient remains still.

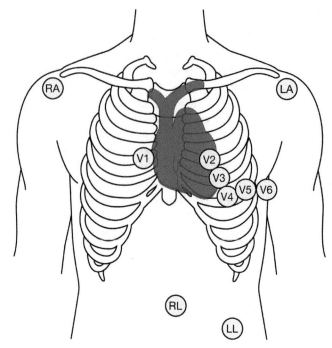

Figure 3.1 12-lead ECG electrode placement.

- When analysing the recording make note of:
  - patient name and date of birth
  - ECG date
  - calibration of recording
  - rate
  - axis
  - rhythm
  - initiation of depolarisation
  - P wave
  - PR interval
  - QRS width
  - QRS height
  - QT interval
  - STR segment
  - T wave
  - U waves.

Cardiac output monitoring

- Measurement of the cardiac output is a fundamental part of managing the critically ill patient.
- Cardiac output is the amount of blood being ejected from the heart each minute. Taken in the clinical context it can be used to make a diagnosis, monitor interventions or guide proactive intervention.
- The application of Ohm's law (V=IR) makes the cardiac output 'flow', the blood pressure is the 'potential difference' and therefore a value for the 'resistance' of the cardiovascular system can be derived. This can be applied to both the systemic and the pulmonary circulations.
- As a key determinant of oxygen delivery, cardiac output can be used to estimate oxygen transport to and from the tissues globally.
- It is beyond the scope of this book to look at the many physiological and paraphysiological (mathematical derivative) values that can be produced using techniques of measuring output and their many applications.
- The method of deriving output is traditionally by a dilution technique. A dye at known concentration is injected into the circulation over a short time period, and the rate of the initial climb and then decline in concentration during a circulation time will indicate the volume of dilution.
- With the pulmonary artery catheter, dye is injected into the right atrium and the concentration in the pulmonary artery is measured continuously. The quantity of dye divided by the area under the dilution/concentration curve will give the cardiac output (Stewart-Hamilton equation). Indocyanine green was once the dye used, but in more recent times saline at low temperature is more common. The temperature is measured by a thermistor in the pulmonary artery. It is reasonably accurate and reproducible, using water or saline, but is affected by many factors such as cardiac rhythm and the phase of ventilation.
- The pulmonary artery catheter is invasive and new less invasive methods are increasing in popularity.
- Pulse contour analysis of arterial waveforms can be used to estimate cardiac output.
  - The PiCCO is a calibrated pulse contour method. A catheter is placed in a large artery and the waveform monitored. A modified dye dilution technique is used with cold fluid injected into a central line and temperature measured at the artery. This is then used to calibrate the pulse contour.
  - The LIDCO is similar but uses a single dose of lithium to do the dilution and calibrate the pulse contour analysis. It usually works using a more peripheral artery.
  - Both of these methods use an algorithm based on pulse contour analysis to measure cardiac output. Both can be recalibrated, and this should be done regularly. The more peripheral the artery the more susceptible it is to changing physiological circumstances; this may render the previous calibration inappropriate for ongoing use and necessitate recalibration. In real terms they work reasonably well most of the time.
  - Newer devices use pulse contour analyses based on population- or general physiology-based algorithms, hence needing no calibration. These tend to work under a wide range of relatively normal circumstances but become less reliable at extremes of cardiac output.

- ○ An even newer device uses a pressure recording analytical method, PRAM. This derives extremely accurate values for cardiac output from the pressure wave form of a peripheral artery. It does not need calibrating and uses a sophisticated algorithm to derive beat-to-beat stroke volume estimations.
- ○ The obvious advantage of these methods is their simplicity and safety but this is balanced against the accuracy of the estimations, which are uncalibrated. Clearly, variability in arterial compliance and in changing vasomotor tone must be built into the algorithm if they are to be reliable. How accurate they need to be for clinical practice is debatable, and as monitors of 'trends' they are probably very useful.
- The oesophageal Doppler measures cardiac output using a flexible ultrasound probe, inserted orally or nasally into the oesophagus. Due to the close anatomical proximity of the oesophagus to the aorta, there is minimal signal interference from bone, soft tissue, and lung. Blood flow velocity in the descending aorta is measured directly and when combined with the calculated aortic cross-sectional area, haemodynamic variables including stroke volume and cardiac output can be calculated.
- Cardiac output can also be measured using transthoracic impedance, measured through externally applied electrodes. Impedance changes with the cardiac cycle due to changes in blood volume. The rate of change of impedance relates to cardiac output.

Intra-abdominal pressure measurement

Indications

- Suspected abdominal compartment syndrome.
- Where a significant rise in intra-abdominal pressure might take place. Some newer invasive abdominal endoscopic procedures can result in high intraperitoneal pressures.

Contraindications

- None

Complications

- Inaccurate measurements

Equipment

- Needle
- Pressure transducer system
  - Provides a continuous column of fluid between cannula and transducer
  - 500 ml bag 0.9% saline
  - 'Pressure bag' to pressurize saline bag to 300 mmHg
- Electrical monitor to provide a digital value or waveform

Sites

- Via the injection port on the urinary catheter

Insertion technique

- Set up pressure transducer system
- Attach needle to end of system ensuring that all air has been expelled from line
- 'Zero' the system
- Insert needle, in sterile manner, into injection port of urinary catheter
- Clamp urinary catheter

Important points/cautions

- This is not a direct measurement and is prone to inaccuracies.
- The pressure being measured is the intra-vesical pressure and not a direct measurement of intra-abdominal pressure. Any measurement taken should be assessed along with other clinical indications of raised intra-abdominal pressure (abdominal girth, renal function, bowel function and overall clinical state) and focus should be on the trend rather than the absolute value.

Arterial blood gas sampling

Indications

- Analysis of respiratory and metabolic disorders

Contraindications

- Absolute:
  - none.
- Relative:
  - local sepsis
  - coagulopathy.

Complications

- Haematoma:
  - Limit with firm pressure for 3 minutes
- Dissection
- Thrombosis
- Aneurysm formation

Equipment

- Sterile swab (alcohol or chlorhexidine)
- Local anaesthetic:
  - Lidocaine 1% **without** adrenaline (epinephrine)
- Heparinized 2 ml syringe:
  - Pre-prepared by manufacturer
  - Normal 2 ml syringe with 23G needle
  - Draw heparin up (1000 U/ml) and expel so only enough remains to coat the walls.
- Ice for transportation:
  - Unless point of care analyser available
- Assistant to provide pressure on puncture site

Sites

- Radial artery:
  - Preferred site as easily accessible, superficial and collateral circulation
- Femoral artery
- Brachial artery (less common)
- Dorsalis pedis artery (less common)
- Posterior tibial artery (less common)

Technique (for radial artery sample)

- Hyperextend wrist.
  - A 500 ml bag of fluid works well.
  - Tape forearm +/- hand to an arm board or ask assistant to help hold in position.
- Clean skin thoroughly.
- Infiltrate local anaesthetic over point of insertion and massage to avoid distorting anatomy.
- Hold syringe like a pencil and insert through skin at a 30- to 45-degree angle to skin surface.
- Advance needle, gently aspirating.

- Arterial blood will be bright red and may push plunger back (especially in commercially available syringes with lower plunger resistance).
- Collect about 2 ml blood.
- Remove needle from artery and apply pressure to puncture site for 3-5 minutes or until bleeding stops.
- Expel air and apply cap to syringe.
- If blood gas analysis is to be delayed by more than 2 minutes it is important to expel all air bubbles or froth to avoid inaccurate pO_2 and pCO_2 measurement (C K Biswas et al.).
  - If the delay is likely to be longer than this then it is recommended that the sample be stored at a cool temperature, again to avoid inaccurate measurements, and this can be achieved by storing the sample in ice (Nanji et al.).

Important points/cautions

- In a hypotensive peripherally collapsed patient arterial puncture and then pressure may result in thrombosis. If in doubt use a larger artery.
- Pressure may need to be applied for longer than 3 minutes in presence of coagulopathy.
- Watch for haematoma formation.

Tips and advice

- If no obvious arterial puncture is achieved on insertion, withdraw needle slowly while gently aspirating. Occasionally the needle will have passed through the artery without aspiration of blood and by withdrawing slowly arterial blood may be aspirated on needle removal.
- It is often best to re-angle the needle through the original puncture point than to completely remove the needle when no puncture is achieved on first pass. Be methodical in locating the artery rather than repeating punctures in different locations.

References/further reading

Biswas CK, Ramos JM, Agroyannis B and Kerr DN (1982). Blood gas analysis: effect of air bubbles in syringe and delay in estimation. *British Medical Journal (Clin Res Ed)* 27 p. 923–927.
Nanji AA and Whitlow KJ (1984). Is it necessary to transport arterial blood samples on ice for pH and gas analysis? *Canadian Journal of Anaesthesia* 31 p. 568–71.

Chapter 4
Airway Procedures

Airway maintenance

- Maintaining a patent airway is a core skill for anaesthetists and intensive care staff.
- Establishing a patent airway is **always** the starting point for resuscitation attempts and assessment of the critically ill (as in ABC).
- Many indications:
  - during general anaesthesia for surgical procedures
  - in critically ill patients
  - in trauma (especially facial injuries and head injuries)
  - in patients with decreased conscious level
  - in sedated patients
  - in obese people (obstructive sleep apnoea)
  - many more…

Positioning

Indications

- Maintaining a patent airway is a core anaesthetic skill.
- Often, simple changes in patient positioning can open an obstructed airway.

Contraindications

- 'Head tilt, chin lift' must **not** be performed in patients with suspected cervical spine (C-spine) injuries.
- Care with any movement of neck (C-spine) in patients with:
  - trauma victims
  - rheumatoid arthritis
  - ankylosing spondylitis
  - cervical spondylosis/osteoarthritis
  - any condition affecting the neck.

Complications

- Hypoxia secondary to an obstructed airway if manoeuvres fail.
- Risk of C-spine damage and spinal cord injury in susceptible patients.

Equipment

- None needed
- Adjuncts may be useful (see later sections in this chapter)

Technique

- Inspect airway.
- Remove any obvious obstructions **with care**.
- In patients **without** suspected C-spine injury, use 'head tilt, chin lift' (See Figure 4.1).
  - Displaces tongue from back of pharynx.
- In suspected C-spine injuries, use 'jaw thrust' manoeuvre (See Figures 4.2 and 4.3)
  - Maintain manual in-line cervical spine immobilisation at all times
    - Assistance needed

Important points/cautions

- After **every** intervention such as a 'head-tilt' manoeuvre, **reassess** the patient.
  - Ensure that the intervention has had desired effect.

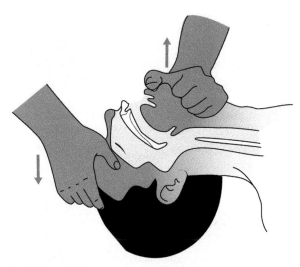

Figure 4.1 Head tilt, chin lift positioning.

○ Observe:
  ■ chest wall movement
  ■ decreased noise when breathing
  ■ improved breath sounds on auscultation
  ■ presence of end-tidal CO_2 (if monitored)
  ■ 'fogging' of masks.
- **If you are unable to maintain a patent airway in a situation where hypoxia may result, call for help immediately.**

Tips and advice
- Simple changes in positioning of the head, jaw, pillow, mask and your hands can often have great effects.

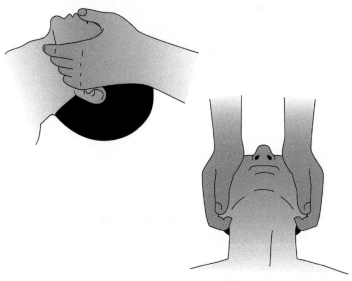

Figure 4.2 Jaw thrust.

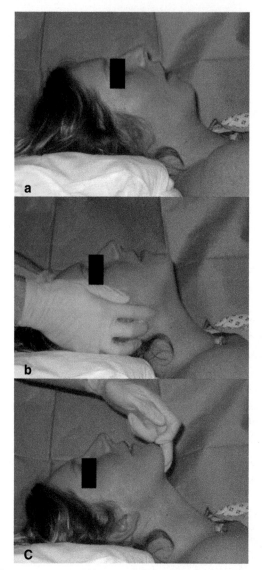

Figure 4.3 Effect of jaw thrust and chin lift/head tilt. a. Anaesthetized, airway unsupported b. Jaw thrust c. Chin lift, head tilt.

- Occasionally turning the patients head slightly to one side will displace the tongue from occluding the larynx.
- Hypoxia kills – always call for help early if you are struggling with an airway.
- Administration of supplemental oxygen should **always** accompany airway optimisation.

Oropharyngeal airway (aka Guedel Airway)

- Anatomically shaped plastic airway

Indications

- To maintain patency of the upper airway.
- Holds tongue and epiglottis forwards.
- Consider using if simple patient-positioning manoeuvres have failed.

Contraindications

- No absolute contraindications
- Caution in facial trauma
- Do not insert if foreign objects, vomitus or copious secretions are in the oral cavity, as the airway can push them further down.

Complications

- Caution in patients with pharyngeal reflexes, as gagging and vomiting could occur.
- Trauma to oral tissues on insertion. These airways must be inserted gently. They will tear mucosa.
- Dental trauma: teeth, caps and crowns can be dislodged.
- Can make obstruction worse, especially if tongue gets pushed in front of airway.

Equipment

- Airways of varying sizes
- Curved portion contains air channel
- Flange at oral end to prevent ingress into mouth
- 'Bite block' sits between teeth
- Choose correct size:
  - airway can be 'sized' by placing one end at the patient's incisors; the other end should just reach the angle of the jaw (mandible)
  - most common sizes for use in adults are 2, 3, and 4 (small, medium and large respectively)
  - smaller airways exist for paediatric use.

Insertion technique

- Choose correct airway (see above).
- Open patient's mouth and ensure no foreign material is present.
- Insert the airway into the mouth in the 'upside-down' position.

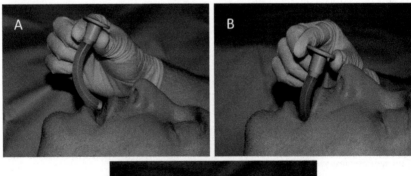

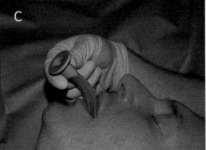

Figure 4.4 Insertion of oropharyngeal airway.

- Insert as far as junction between hard and soft palettes.
- Rotate airway through 180° so it lies in the correct orientation.
- Reapply oxygen mask.
- Reassess the patient.

Important points/cautions

- Insertion technique above helps to avoid pushing the tongue backwards.
- Remove the airway if the patient gags or strains.
- If suspected C-spine injury, maintain alignment and immobilisation.
- Care in patients with bleeding disorders.

Tips and advice

- Positioning manoeuvres such as 'head tilt, chin lift' may be needed in addition to airway insertion.
- Air channel should allow passage of suction catheters.

Nasopharyngeal airway

- Airway inserted into nasopharynx, bypassing mouth and oropharynx.
- Distal end sits above epiglottis and below base of tongue.

Indications

- As for insertion of oropharyngeal airway (see above).
- Better tolerated than oropharyngeal airway in semi-awake patients.
- Consider especially if:
  - mouth cannot be opened (e.g. trauma, trismus)
  - oropharyngeal airway has not relieved obstruction.

Contraindications

- **Do not** use in patients with suspected basal skull fracture **unless** there is no other way to prevent life-threatening hypoxia.
- Caution in patients with:
  - bleeding disorders
  - on anticoagulant medication
  - nasal deformities, polyps, sepsis.

Complications

- Trauma to the nose, nasopharynx and upper airway
- Bleeding (can be profuse) – occurs in 30% of insertions
- 'Loss' of airway into nose (prevented by use of safety pin or flange)
- Creation of false passage
- Can worsen airway obstruction

Equipment

- Nasopharyngeal airways of varying sizes
- Lubricating jelly
- A safety pin (if the nasopharyngeal airway to be used requires one; some newer airways have a large flange at the nasal end and do not need to be used with a pin)

Sites

- Either nostril can be used.
- Nostrils should be examined for obvious obstructions or deformities.
- Clearest nostril should be used.

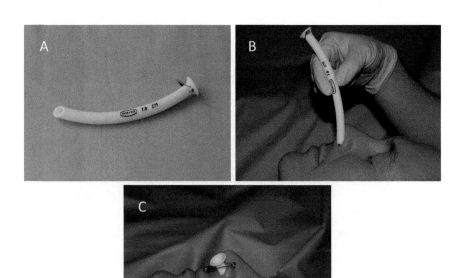

Figure 4.5 Insertion of nasopharyngeal airway.

Insertion technique

- Choose correct size:
  - sized in millimetres (internal diameter)
  - size 6–7 mm suitable for most adults.
- Check patency of nostril to be used.
- Insert safety pin through the flange at the proximal end of the airway (if needed).
- Lubricate the airway with water-soluble jelly.
- Insert bevel end of airway into nostril, with the curve directed to the patient's feet.
- Push **gently** back, in line with floor of nose.
- If **any** obstruction is met, stop and try the other nostril.
- Once in place, **reassess** the patient.

Important points/cautions

- As above.
  - Do **not** force the airway if obstruction is met.
  - Bleeding may be occult and may pass into the airway:
    - suction may be required.
  - Suction is possible through nasopharyngeal airways.

Tips and advice

- Insertion with a slight twisting action may ease passage.
- Chin lift or jaw thrust may still be required.
- Don't forget to reapply the oxygen mask and constantly reassess the patient.

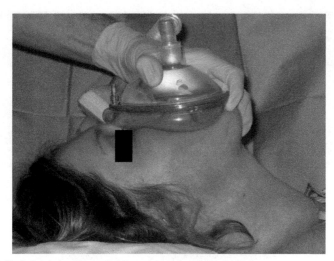

Figure 4.6 Single handed mask ventilation.

Facemasks

- **Always** check the oxygen supply to the mask is patent and functional.
- Facemasks are designed to fit the face anatomically.
  - Newer disposable masks do not always conform easily.
- Many designs exist.

Indications

- Delivery of gases, volatile anaesthetics to patients
- Used in a wide variety of settings, e.g.:
  - resuscitation
  - supplemental oxygen therapy

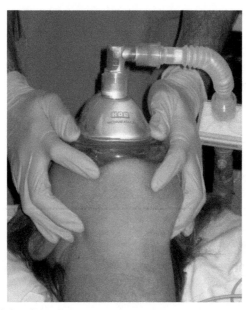

Figure 4.7 Two handed mask ventilation.

- ○ nebulizer administration
- ○ induction and maintenance of anaesthesia
- ○ administration of entonox for analgesia.

Contraindications

- None

Complications

- Dead space may be increased by the internal volume of the mask
  - ○ May be up to 200 ml in adults
  - ○ Of particular importance in children

Equipment

- Appropriate mask in terms of:
  - ○ correct size for the patient's face
  - ○ correct mask for the required use
  - ○ for oxygen delivery, mask type affects maximum percentage that can be delivered.
    - ■ E.g. variable performance masks, Venturi masks (HAFOE masks).
- For induction and maintenance of anaesthesia, and for resuscitation, a bag-valve-mask setup with a tight fitting mask (e.g. Ambu facemask) is used.
  - ○ Delivers high concentrations of oxygen if needed (up to 90%).

Sites

- Face masks usually cover mouth and nose
- Nasal masks are sometimes used; e.g. CPAP for sleep apnoea

Important points/cautions

- Transparent masks are preferred to opaque ones, as this allows visualization of vomitus and secretions.
- Remember that dead-space may be increased by the mask used.
- May be impossible to achieve a good seal against the patient's face due to:
  - ○ facial hair
  - ○ facial deformities
  - ○ secretions.

Tips and advice

- A snug fit is more easily achieved with a mask that has an air-filled cushion applied to the face.
  - ○ Ensure this cuff is inflated adequately.
- Variations in hand-position may be required to achieve a good seal against the face
- Use of two hands on the mask may be necessary.
  - ○ Get an assistant to squeeze the bag if needed.
- Ensure the correct oxygen flow rate is used for the mask in use.
  - ○ E.g. bag-valve-mask systems should have a high flow rate of 10–15 L/min
  - ○ Nebulizers should have a flow rate of 4–6 L/min
  - ○ Venturi masks require different oxygen flow rates depending on the Venturi device used.
- Well-fitting dentures may improve the fit of a facemask, and the resulting seal, if left in place.

Laryngeal mask airways

- Laryngeal mask airways (LMAs) are frequently used supraglottic airways.
- LMAs were invented by Dr. A. Brain in London and were developed at the Royal Berkshire Hospital in 1981 as an alternative to the facemask.
- Many variations on the original LMA theme now exist.

Indications

- Alternative to the facemask for achieving and maintaining airway control during general anaesthesia.
- Airway maintenance in fully starved, anaesthetized patients:
  - **only** if low risk of aspiration
  - if neither anaesthetic technique nor surgery require the patient to have a protected airway with a tracheal tube.
- In resuscitation attempts if a tracheal tube (TT) cannot be placed.
- Airway obstruction in unconscious patients
- As an aid in difficult intubation situations, and failed intubation cases (see later section on difficult airways).

Contraindications

- LMAs sit above the larynx, and therefore offer little or limited protection against aspiration of gastric contents.
  - **Do not** use if a full stomach is suspected
  - **Do not** use if there is a risk of aspiration, including:
    - hiatus hernia
    - gastro-oesophageal reflux
    - certain surgical procedures.
- Morbidly obese patients under general anaesthetic
- >14 weeks pregnant
- Multiple or massive injury
- Acute abdominal or thoracic injury
- Where peak inspiratory pressures may exceed 20–30 cm H_2O
- Patients with low pulmonary compliance

Complications

- Mechanical
  - Failed insertion (0.3–4%)
  - Ineffective seal (<5%)
  - Poor positioning (20–35%)
- Traumatic
  - Local tissue damage to lips, mouth, tongue, pharynx, larynx
  - Sore throat
  - Dysphagia
  - Dysarthria
- Pathophysiological
  - Coughing (<2%)
  - Vomiting (0.02–5%)
  - Regurgitation of gastric contents
  - Aspiration of gastric contents (2.3 per 10,000 insertions)

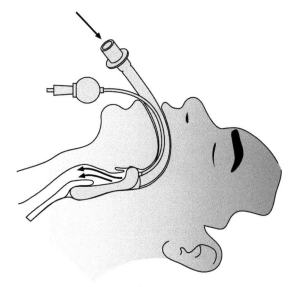

Figure 4.8 Laryngeal mask in place.

Equipment
- Many different types of LMA exist to accommodate varying needs (see Table 4.1).
- All LMAs have:
  - airway tube with standard 15 mm connection
  - mask +/– inflatable cuff
  - inflation line if inflatable cuff present.
- Mask is designed to conform to contours of hypopharynx with lumen facing the laryngeal inlet (see Figure 4.8).
- LMAs are sized from 1 to 6
  - 1 is smallest; 6 is largest
  - Choice of size depends on weight of patient (see Table 4.2)

Sites
- All LMAs are supraglottic airways

Insertion technique
- See Figures 4.9 and 4.10.
- Hold the LMA like a pencil.

Table 4.1 The commonly encountered types of LMA and their uses

Type of LMA	Description
Classic LMA	The original LMA as described above and shown in Figure 4.4
Single use Classic LMA	As above, but disposable after one use
ProSeal LMA	Advanced design. For use with positive pressure ventilation. Allows drainage of stomach via special port
Flexible LMA and single use Flexible LMA	Wire-reinforced, flexible airway tube allowing the tube to be moved without obstructing or moving the mask
Intubating LMA	Facilitates intubation via the LMA with a specific endotracheal tube
Ctrach LMA	Intubating LMA with integrated fibreoptic system to aid intubation

Table 4.2 Sizing of LMAs

LMA Airway Size	Patient Size	Max. Cuff Inflation Volumes (ml of air)
1	Up to 5 kg	4
1.5	5–10 kg	7
2	10–20 kg	10
2.5	20–30 kg	14
3	30–50 kg	20
4	50–70 kg	30
5	70–100 kg	40
6	>100kg	50

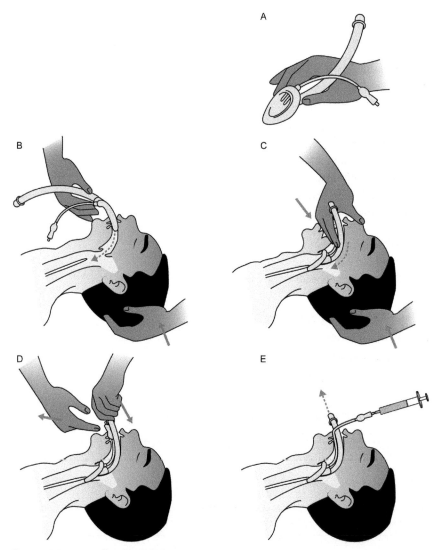

Figure 4.9 Insertion of laryngeal mask airway.

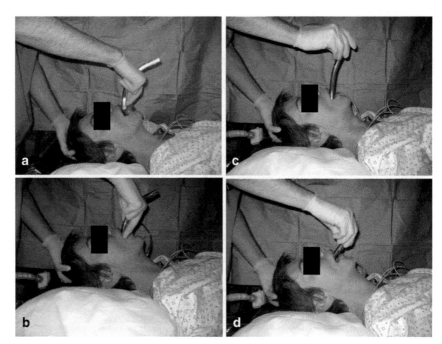

Figure 4.10 Insertion of a laryngeal mask airway.

- Press the mask up against the hard palate.
- Slide the mask inward, keeping it pressed against hard palate with extended index finger.
- Push the index finger towards the back of the patient's mouth.
- Advance the LMA until resistance is felt.
- Hold the outer end of the airway tube while the index finger is withdrawn.
- Inflate the cuff with the appropriate volume of air.
- Connect to breathing circuit and check airway is patent.
- Insert a bite block if the LMA doesn't have one integrated.
- Securely fix the LMA in place (tape and tie).

Important points/cautions

- As above, ensure LMA is appropriate for situation.
- Ensure your own safety when inserting a finger into patient's mouth:
  - wear gloves
  - ensure patient is deeply anaesthetized.
- The LMA can obstruct the airway if it does not sit in a good position.
- There must be easy flow both in and out and no clinical signs of obstruction such as tugging etc.
- Securely fix the LMA as it can easily be dislodged.

Tips and advice

- 'Sniffing the morning air' positioning of the head may aid insertion.
- Having an assistant perform a jaw thrust may aid insertion.
- Lubricating the outside of the mask may be useful.

- Insertion with the cuff partially inflated may aid insertion.
- Use of a laryngoscope blade may aid placement in exceptional circumstances.
- When in the correct position, the neck will swell around the thyroid and cricoid area when the cuff is inflated.
- On cuff inflation, the tube will move out of the mouth somewhat – this is normal.
- The ProSeal LMA comes with an introducer which may aid insertion.
- A fibreoptic scope pre-loaded with an endotracheal tube can be passed via an LMA in some cases of difficult intubation.
- Not every LMA will be anatomically suited to every patient.

Tracheal intubation

Oral tracheal intubation

- Core anaesthetic/intensive care skill
- Passing a tracheal tube through the mouth into the trachea
- Useful in elective and emergency situations

Indications

- Emergencies, where intubation facilitates oxygenation and positive pressure ventilation
- Inability to protect the airway
  - Decreased conscious level (Glasgow Coma Score <8)
  - Excessive intraoral secretions that cannot be spontaneously cleared
  - Absent gag reflex (e.g. CVA, neuromuscular disorders)
  - Bleeding that may jeopardize the airway
- Elective intubation in many circumstances
  - Limited access to the airway (e.g. neurosurgery)
  - When maintenance of the airway may be difficult
  - 'Shared airway' when surgeon and anaesthetist both need access to the airway (e.g. ENT, head and neck surgery)
  - Prone patients
  - When positive pressure ventilation is indicated, especially when sustained for long periods
    - Can be performed via a LMA but lower pressure limits apply
  - When accurate control of ventilation is required
    - Thoracic surgery
    - Neurosurgery

Contraindications

- Few contraindications exist.
- Known laryngeal problems (relative).
  - E.g. carcinoma, obstructive lesions
- Caution and senior help needed with the following.
  - Potential/previous difficult intubation
  - Full stomach or potential for full stomach
  - Specific problems which may hamper vision
    - Gastrointestinal bleeding
    - Upper airway bleeding
  - Other factors
    - Trauma (C-spine, maxillofacial)
    - Caesarean section
    - Extremes of age
    - Medical conditions, intercurrent illnesses

Complications

- Failure to intubate
  - Potentially fatal if unable to maintain oxygenation via other means
- Hypoxia if intubation attempt is prolonged
- Autonomic stimulation

- ○ Vagal
  - ■ Bradycardia
  - ○ Sympathetic
  - ■ Tachycardia, hypertension
- Trauma from laryngoscope blade or from tube itself
  - ○ Lips, mouth, teeth, tongue, pharynx, larynx, vocal cords, trachea
  - ○ Surgical emphysema may result
  - ○ Pneumothorax
  - ○ **Care with dental implants, caps, crowns**
- Bronchospasm and laryngospasm
- Endobronchial intubation
  - ○ More often enters right main bronchus for anatomical reasons (right main bronchus comes off carina at less acute angle than left)
- Tracheal stenosis
  - ○ Usually after prolonged periods with tube in situ
- Recurrent laryngeal nerve injury
- Laryngoscopy can cause cervical subluxation in susceptible patients

Equipment

- The following is just a guide, and different situations may necessitate more equipment, or more specialized apparatus.
- **All** equipment to be used **must** be checked prior to starting (**this is not optional!**). The margin of safety is narrow.
  - ○ Two laryngoscopes (see Figure 4.11)
    - ■ With different size blades

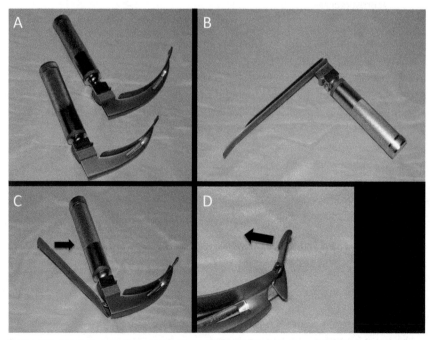

Figure 4.11 Laryngoscopes. a) Macintosh blades; b) Straight blade; and c and d) McCoy blade.

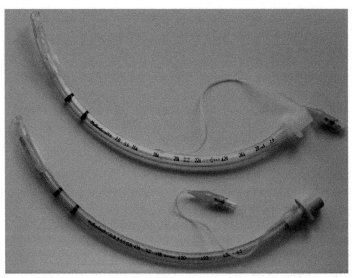

Figure 4.12 Tracheal tubes.

- Macintosh blades 3 and 4 usually suffice for most adults
- Straight blades may be needed for children
- Consider McCoy blades for potentially difficult intubation (seek senior assistance)
  ○ Endotracheal tubes (see Figure 4.12).
    - One of the appropriate size
    - One a size smaller than anticipated
    - For children, one smaller and one larger than calculated size, 0.5 mm increments
  ○ Appropriate connections
    - Filters, catheter mount, breathing circuit
  ○ Syringe to inflate cuff (usually 10–20 ml syringe)
  ○ Lubricating jelly (water-based)
  ○ Oxygen supply
  ○ Suction
  ○ Self-inflating bag with appropriate mask
  ○ Gum elastic bougie
  ○ Minimum monitoring
    - See section on monitoring
  ○ A skilled assistant, though not essential for every intubation, is certainly helpful.
- In addition to the above, a method of maintaining anaesthesia or sedation must be available if the patient's conscious level before intubation mandates it.
- Usual sizes for endotracheal tubes:
  ○ Adult female–7.0 mm internal diameter
  ○ Adult male–8.0 mm internal diameter
  ○ Larger and smaller adults may require different size tubes, and the above is only a guide.

- ○ Paediatric use – tube size is roughly calculated using:
  - ■ (AGE/4) + 4–4.5 mm (for > 1 year)
  - ■ For children < 1 year:

Weight/Age	Tube size (internal diameter in mm)
> 2 kg	2.5
2–4 kg	3.0
Term neonate	3.5
3–12 months	4.0

- ○ Uncuffed tubes for < 10 years
  - ■ This is NOT an absolute rule, and with modern cuff design, many institutions are using cuffed tubes in much younger children
- ○ **As a guide**, tube insertion depth is calculated as follows:
  - ■ (AGE/2) + 12 (for > 1 year)
  - ■ For < 1 year:
    - 0–3 months–10 cm (at lips)
    - 3–6 months–11 cm
    - 6–12 months–12 cm

Sites

- ● Intubation can be performed in any way that results in a tube being situated in the trachea. The commonest sites are:
  - ○ oral–commonest route
  - ○ nasal–see later section, this chapter.

Insertion technique

- ● See Figure 4.13.
- ● All of the equipment listed above should be at hand and checked.
- ● Remove patient's dentures if present.
- ● Ensure the patient is well oxygenated (see later section on rapid sequence induction).
- ● Induce anaesthesia and give muscle relaxant if indicated.
- ● Position patient's head in the 'sniffing the morning air' position.
  - ○ Neck flexed, head extended.
  - ○ A pillow is almost universally essential (**not** in young children who have relatively large heads).
  - ○ See Figure 4.14.
- ● Hold laryngoscope in **left** hand (even if right handed).
- ● Introduce the blade of the laryngoscope **carefully** into the **right** side of the mouth, avoiding contact with the teeth and lips.
- ● 'Sweep' the tongue to left of mouth with the blade.
- ● Gently advance the blade behind the tongue **(never** force the blade)
- ● Place the tip of the laryngoscope blade in the valecula (in front of the epiglottis) **or** behind the epiglottis if using a straight bladed laryngoscope.
- ● **Do not** use the laryngoscope as a lever, but lift it away from you
- ● Lift tongue, soft tissues and jaw forward.
- ● View the vocal cords and laryngeal inlet (see Figures 4.15 and 4.16).

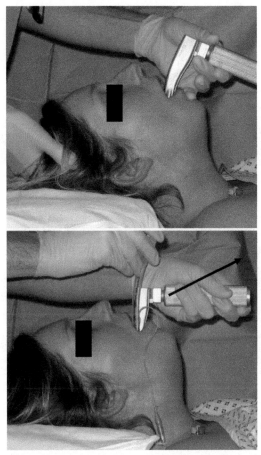

Figure 4.13 Tracheal intubation. a. Note positioning – Neck flexed, head extended. Use a finger, or ask an assistant, to pull down the lower lip to aid insertion. An alternative technique uses the right hand to open the mouth wide using thumb and middle finger. b. Arrow indicates the direction of force applied to the laryngoscope.

- Pass the tube through the cords with your right hand until the cuff sits below them.
- Inflate the cuff with just enough air to prevent leakage.
  - Cuff pressure should not exceed 30 cmH$_2$O.
- Attach tube to breathing circuit.
- Test to ensure correct position (ensure somebody holds onto the tube during this period).
  - You should have seen the tube pass between vocal cords (gold standard).
  - End-tidal CO$_2$ (E$_T$CO$_2$) should be seen on capnograph/capnometer.
  - Oesophageal detector (if available).
  - Chest should rise on inflation.
  - Auscultate both sides of chest and epigastrium.
  - Patient should remain pink and have good oxygenation on monitoring.
  - Consider requesting a CXR (ICU, trauma, emergency intubation).
- **If there is any doubt about the position of the tube then remove it and oxygenate the patient.**

A

B

C

D

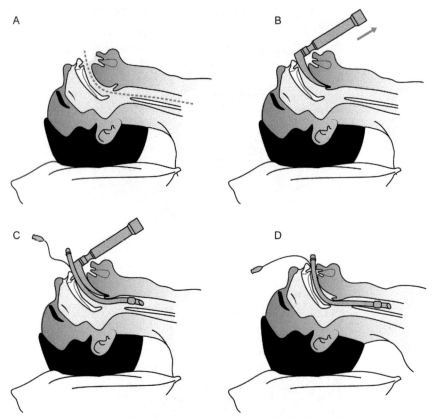

Figure 4.14 'Sniffing the morning air' position and laryngoscopy diagrams.

- **'If in doubt take it out'**
- Once correct position is confirmed, securely fix the tube. Tie, tapes, fixation devices can all be used.

Important points/cautions

- Remember to **always** to check equipment prior to use.
- Patients should be fasted for **at least** 6 hours for solid food and **at least** 2 hours for clear fluids.

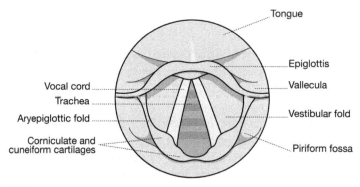

Tongue

Epiglottis

Vallecula

Vocal cord

Vestibular fold

Trachea

Aryepiglottic fold

Corniculate and cuneiform cartilages

Piriform fossa

Figure 4.15 View at laryngoscopy.

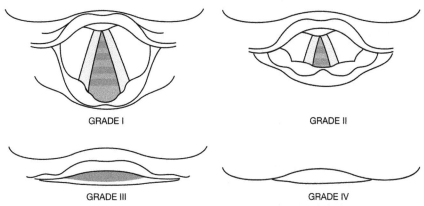

GRADE I   GRADE II

GRADE III   GRADE IV

Figure 4.16 Cormack and Lehane Grades.

- Correct positioning of the patient's head is important and can markedly improve chances of intubation.
- Call for help **early** if running into difficulties.
  - Hypoxia can kill
  - Repeated intubation attempts can be very dangerous and traumatic.

Tips and advice

- Always have in mind a backup plan for an unanticipated difficult intubation and know the drill for a failed intubation (see later section).
  - Where will help come from?
  - Who will go and get help?
  - What will you do whilst awaiting help?
- Preparation (equipment, drugs, assistance, environment, breathing circuit, and patient) will help to avoid complications.
- Keep an eye on the time taken for an intubation attempt.
  - If SpO_2 starts to fall, then stop, oxygenate, call for help and reattempt.
- Many things can improve an initially poor view at laryngoscopy.
  - Change position of head, height of bed, add or remove pillow.
  - Use of different laryngoscope blades:
    - longer or shorter Macintosh blade
    - McCoy blade
    - straight blade (esp. younger children)
    - polio blade (pregnancy, obese, large breasts)
    - short laryngoscope handle, with any of above blades.
  - Application of cricoid pressure or BURP (backwards, upwards, to-the-right pressure) by an assistant.
  - Suctioning of secretions.
- Use of adjuncts may aid passage of tube.
  - Bougies (see later).
  - Introducers/stylets.

Nasal intubation

- Useful in elective and emergency anaesthesia
- Useful in intensive care, especially in neonates/paediatrics

Indications

- Three sets of indications.
  - Oral surgical procedures:
    - where LMA cannot be used
    - where an oral ETT would affect the surgical field.
  - Situations where mouth-opening is markedly reduced, making oral intubation difficult or impossible.
    - Trismus:
      - trauma (e.g. fracture of mandible)
      - infections (abscesses, tetanus)
      - congenital deformities.
    - Facial trauma with deformity:
      - **beware** possible basal skull fracture.
  - Where patient comfort and tolerance is a factor
    - Long-term intubation (tracheostomy more common in this situation)
    - Awake intubation techniques

Contraindications

- None are absolute, but the benefits of nasal intubation would have to outweigh the risks.
  - Basal skull fracture
  - Coagulopathy or anticoagulant therapy
  - Epiglottitis
  - Nasal sepsis
    - Can lead to intracranial infection
  - Nasal obstruction or deformity
    - Polyps, septal deformities or nasal trauma
  - Midface instability

Complications

- As for oral intubation (see above), plus the following.
  - Nasal bleeding:
    - may be profuse
    - may require ENT input
    - may be concealed at first.
  - Trauma to nose and nasopharynx.
  - Creation of false passages in nose.
  - Nasal/sinus sepsis in long-term intubated.
  - Trauma to adenoids, especially in children.

Equipment

- As for oral intubation (see above).
- Again, **check all equipment prior to starting**
- In addition to equipment for oral intubation:
  - correct size of tube for NASAL intubation
    - As for oral tubes in paediatric use

- ▪ In adults, usually size 6–6.5 for most patients
- ▪ Occasionally use larger or smaller tubes
  - ○ specially designed nasal tubes may be used (see later section on special airways)
  - ○ vasoconstrictors and local anaesthesia may be needed prior to intubation
    - ▪ phenylephrine, cocaine or Moffat's solution, lidocaine
  - ○ Magill forceps.

Sites
- ● Right or left nostril.
- ● Knowledge of anatomy is essential as there is always a 'blind' component to this procedure as the tube passes through the nose and nasopharynx.

Insertion technique (in the anaesthetized patient)
- ● Examine the patient's nose **before** inducing anaesthesia.
  - ○ See which nostril it is easier to breathe through.
  - ○ Ask about any nasal problems.
  - ○ Inspect the nose and nostrils.
- ● Vasoconstrictors (if indicated) can be applied before or after induction of anaesthesia.
- ● Begin once the patient is anaesthetized and well oxygenated.
  - ○ Position as for oral intubation ('sniffing the morning air').
  - ○ Lubricate the distal end of the tube.
  - ○ Introduce the tube into the chosen nostril.
  - ○ The path of insertion is parallel to the palate:
    - ▪ in supine patient this equals vertically downwards
    - ▪ no force should be used; it is a gentle procedure.
  - ○ If resistance is encountered, do not force the tube:
    - ▪ withdraw slightly and angle slightly cephalad
    - ▪ usually this is due to tube hitting inferior concha.
  - ○ Once the tube is felt to pass through the nose:
    - ▪ insert laryngoscope into mouth, as for oral intubation
    - ▪ look for distal end of tube in pharynx
    - ▪ if **not** visible, then advance tube further through nose
    - ▪ once visible, pick up Magill forceps with right hand
    - ▪ insert Magill forceps into mouth
    - ▪ grasp distal end of tube with forceps
    - ▪ advance tube towards and through vocal cords into trachea.
  - ○ Connect the tube to the breathing circuit.
  - ○ Inflate the cuff until leak just disappears.
  - ○ Confirm correct position of tube (see oral intubation section, above).
  - ○ Securely fix the tube in place.
    - ▪ Usually tapes to nose, face and sometimes forehead.

Important points/cautions
- ● Depth of insertion is based on clinical examination in adults.
  - ○ Ensure bilateral air entry
  - ○ Visible passage through cords
  - ○ Bronchoscopic confirmation of position (i.e. looking through tube)

- Depth in paediatrics can be calculated by:
  - (AGE/2) + 15 (for > 1 year)
  - In < 1 year:
    - no formulae exist
    - clinical examination to confirm correct position.

Tips and advice

- Don't cut the tube to be used as this may result in a tube which is too short to pass into the trachea.
- Vasoconstrictors may be very useful.
  - Take care if using topical cocaine preparations, as overdose is possible.
- Magill forceps do not always need to be used to manoeuvre tube into trachea.
  - Tube may sometimes be easily passed through vocal cords just by manipulation of the patient's head and the tube at the nose, or with cricoid pressure.
- Blind nasal intubation used to be practised widely.
  - Depends on skill and experience of operator.
  - May cause unnecessary trauma to airway.
  - Direct vision of tube passing between vocal cords is best way to confirm correct tube placement.
- Ensure tube is securely fastened in position.
  - Especially in surgery where head and face are distant and covered.
  - Movements of the head may more easily move a nasal tube.

Bougies and other intubation aids

- Bougies and other intubation aids should be readily available for all intubation episodes.
- They can greatly increase chances of successful intubation in many circumstances.
- See also later section on difficult intubations.

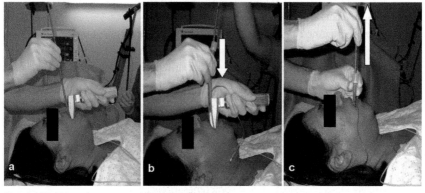

Figure 4.17 Using a bougie to assist tracheal intubation.

Main adjuncts summarized in the following table.

Table 4.3 Intubation adjuncts and their indications

Adjunct	Indications/Uses/Notes
Gum elastic bougie	• difficulty seeing cords • difficulty directing tube towards cords • bougie is passed through cords and tube railroaded over it • never force a bougie
Introducer	• stiffer than bougie • inserted into tube prior to passage • used to adjust curvature of tube • associated with mucosal and other tissue damage
Endotrol tube	• ring-pull on inner curvature • when ring-pull pulled, curvature increases • can be used to direct tube through cords
Bite guards	• protect upper dentition from damage
Local anaesthetic spray	• can prevent coughing • decreases stimulus of intubation • usually lidocaine
Magill forceps	• many uses • directing tubes (esp. nasal) • placing throat packs • removing foreign bodies
Throat pack	• ribbon gauze, moistened • inserted after intubation • placed around tube, above larynx • aims to absorb/catch secretions or blood • prevents soiling of the airway
Retrograde intubation set	• used in difficult intubations • especially in conditions obscuring laryngeal inlet e.g. airway tumours • guidewire introduced through cannula placed through cricothyroid membrane • guidewire directed cephalad, to pass through vocal cords from below • wire grasped in airway by second operator performing laryngoscopy • guiding catheter or tube can be passed over wire, into trachea

Rapid sequence induction (RSI)

- Rapid sequence induction (RSI) is a core anaesthetic skill.
- RSI aims to prevent aspiration of gastric contents during intubation.
- RSI results in a cuffed, tracheal tube in the trachea with the cuff inflated.

Indications

- **Any** situation where the patient may have a full stomach
  - Trauma, opiates and other medications, stress, pain, and diabetes (all can delay gastric emptying)
  - Hiatus hernia or symptomatic gastro-oesophageal reflux
  - Pharyngeal pouch
  - Oesophageal strictures
  - Peritonitis
  - Ileus
  - Bowel obstruction
  - Gastric carcinoma
  - Pyloric stenosis
  - Pregnancy (after 14 weeks gestation)
  - Decreased conscious level
  - Alcohol ingestion
  - Poor historian
  - Inadequate fasting period but surgery/intubation cannot be delayed

Contraindications

- A 'textbook' rapid sequence induction may not always be appropriate:
  - e.g. 'suxamethonium apnoea' or history of malignant hyperthermia where use of suxamethonium would be contraindicated
  - alternative drugs would need to be used (e.g. rocuronium).
- In situations where a difficult intubation is very likely or in specific situations such as epiglottitis, facial trauma or bleeding tonsils, an inhalational induction may be considered.
  - Laryngoscopy performed when patient deeply anaesthetized.
  - Tube passed during spontaneous ventilation.
  - Muscle relaxation administered after tube positioned in trachea.
  - Patient should be in left lateral, head-down position or supine with cricoid pressure applied when deep enough.
- An alternative technique when a difficult intubation is anticipated is an awake fibreoptic intubation (see later section).
  - Fibreoptic scope with endotracheal tube loaded over it.
  - Tube placed under direct vision with patient awake.
  - Local anaesthesia to nose.

Complications

- As for oral intubation (see previous section).
- Additional complications:
  - reactions to induction agent/muscle relaxant
  - 'suxamethonium apnoea' where suxamethonium has greatly prolonged duration of action

○ failure to intubate +/– ventilate

○ aspiration of gastric contents.

Equipment

- As for oral intubation (see previous section).
- All equipment should be checked.
- Appropriate drugs for a rapid sequence induction should be drawn up and checked.
  ○ The 'traditional' RSI involves administration of:
    ■ a sleep dose (usually 5–7 mg/kg) of thiopentone
    ■ 1–2 mg/kg suxamethonium.
  ○ Alternatives exist, and can be used in a modified RSI.
  ○ Emergency drugs should be drawn up, checked and readily available.
    ■ Atropine, glycopyrrolate, and ephedrine, with or without further vasoconstrictor e.g. metaraminol.
- In addition, certain **essential** equipment should be readily available for every rapid sequence induction.
  ○ Patient **must** be on a tipping trolley or table.
  ○ At least one skilled assistant should be present:
    ■ competent at applying cricoid pressure
    ■ to assist in turning patient if regurgitation occurs
    ■ to obtain additional equipment as needed.
  ○ High-volume suction switched on and within reach of the anaesthetist's hand.
  ○ A tight-fitting facemask connected to a breathing circuit capable of delivering high concentrations of oxygen.
  ○ An intravenous cannula in situ with fluids flowing through it.

Sites

- RSI usually involves oral intubation; however, the nasal route could also be used.

Insertion technique

- Once all equipment, drugs and personnel are ready and the patient has given informed consent, the RSI can begin.
- **If there is any possibility of a difficult intubation then seek senior help before starting.**
- Preoxygenate the patient for three minutes:
  ○ use tight fitting facemask connected to high-flow oxygen
  ○ **do not** break the seal of mask on face at all during the three minutes, unless the patient actively vomits
  ○ aim is to fill the functional residual capacity (FRC) with oxygen
  ○ in otherwise healthy, compliant patients three to five maximal inspiratory breaths can achieve similar washout of nitrogen from the FRC
  ○ this 'reserve' of oxygen can 'buy time' in the event of a difficult intubation.
- Once preoxygenation is complete, induce anaesthesia. Usually this is administration of intravenous thiopentone and suxamethonium, as described earlier in this section.
- As the patient is anaesthetized, the assistant should apply cricoid pressure (see important points/cautions).
- Laryngoscopy should take place once the fasciculations (seen with suxamethonium administration) have stopped.

- ○ If fasciculations are not seen (elderly patients, poor muscle mass) then a period of 30–60 seconds should elapse before laryngoscopy is performed.
  - ○ During this period, the seal between facemask and face should not be broken.
  - ○ The patient should **not** be ventilated during this time.
- Perform laryngoscopy as previously described.
- Once the vocal cords are visualized then the tube should be passed into the trachea and the cuff inflated.
- Once the tube is confirmed to be in the correct position (see earlier) then (and **only** then) the cricoid pressure can be released.
- Secure the tube in position.
- Continue anaesthesia as planned.
- If difficulties are encountered in getting a good view during laryngoscopy then it is vital to maintain oxygenation.
  - ○ Anyone undertaking RSIs should be familiar with a failed intubation drill.
  - ○ The Difficult Airway Society (DAS) produces guidelines and algorithms for what to do in the event of failed intubation and in a 'can't intubate, can't ventilate' scenario (see www.das.uk.com).
- The guidelines for a failed RSI (in a non-obstetric adult patient) are reproduced below, with permission.
- Any problems during laryngoscopy: **call for help**
- If poor view:
  - ○ reduce or modify cricoid pressure
  - ○ use a bougie
  - ○ consider alternative laryngoscope.
- No more than three attempts at intubation should be attempted, whilst maintaining:
  - ○ oxygenation with facemask
  - ○ cricoid pressure
  - ○ anaesthesia
    - ▪ boluses of induction agent.
- If unsuccessful, this is a **failed intubation**.
  - ○ Maintain 30 N cricoid force.
  - ○ Use facemask and bag to ventilate:
    - ▪ two person technique
    - ▪ oral/nasal airway
    - ▪ consider reducing cricoid force if ventilation difficult.
- If SpO_2 < 90% with 100% oxygen via facemask, this is **failed oxygenation**.
  - ○ Insert LMA (reduce cricoid force during insertion)
  - ○ Ventilate and oxygenate
  - ○ Maintain anaesthesia
  - ○ If this succeeds in oxygenating patient:
    - ▪ postpone surgery and awaken patient if possible
    - ▪ if in **life-threatening** condition then continue anaesthesia with LMA or ProSeal LMA.
- If SpO_2 still < 90%, then this is **failed ventilation and oxygenation.**
  - ○ 'Rescue' techniques:
    - ▪ cannula cricothyroidotomy (see later section)

- surgical cricothyroidotomy (see later section)
- after above and successful oxygenation, then proceed to a definitive airway as soon as possible
- maintain anaesthesia.

Important points/cautions

- Remember, patients should be fasted for 6 hours for solids and 2 hours for clear fluids, otherwise they have a full stomach.
- In trauma patients, the time between the last meal and the **traumatic incident** itself is a better indicator of the degree of gastric emptying than the period of fasting.
  - It is not uncommon to encounter vomiting up to 24 hours after food ingestion in trauma patients where the trauma occurred shortly after a meal.
- Cricoid pressure (Sellick's manoeuvre) is applied in a particular way, and the assistant at an RSI should be competent and happy to perform this procedure.
  - Use thumb and forefinger of one hand.
  - Pressure on the cricoid cartilage:
    - force of around 10 N in an awake patient, increasing to 30N as anaesthesia deepens
    - force directed backwards in midline
    - cricoid cartilage forms complete ring around trachea and therefore compresses the oesophagus behind the cricoid and the vertebral column.
  - Pressure should only be released under the following circumstances:
    - patient actively vomits
    - once the tube is in the trachea and the anaesthetist asks the assistant to remove the cricoid pressure
    - if a 'can't intubate, can't ventilate' situation has arisen
      - sometimes the removal of the cricoid pressure facilitates ventilation.
  - Modified RSI is any technique which deviates from the 'text book' RSI described above, using thiopentone and suxamethonium.
    - The usual modification is to replace thiopentone with an induction dose of another agent, such as propofol.
    - Rocuronium (non-depolarising, longer acting muscle relaxant) is gaining popularity as a replacement for suxamethonium in RSIs.
      - Dose of 0.9 mg/kg needed.
      - Good intubating conditions in around 60 seconds.
      - Can now be rapidly reversed using sugammadex in the event of a failed intubation.

Tips and advice

- It is important to consider whether surgery can be postponed until the patient is fully starved, as RSI is not without risk.
  - Close liaison and discussion with surgical team essential
  - Consider alternatives:
    - regional anaesthesia
    - local anaesthesia.
- Familiarity with a 'text book' RSI technique is essential before attempting to modify the procedure.

- Comprehensive preparation is essential.
- Insertion and aspiration of a naso-gastric tube may be of use in certain situations, to reduce the risk of regurgitation. This does not replace the need for a RSI though
- Pre-medication may be of use in certain situations:
  - usually only in elective situations in patients with reflux or hiatus hernia
  - antacids – e.g. sodium citrate, in pregnant patients
  - PPIs or H_2 antagonists (decrease gastric acid secretion)
  - metoclopramide 10mg, to increase lower-oesophageal sphincter tone.
- Ensure the patient is fully informed about RSI.
  - Cricoid pressure can be frightening if applied to an unsuspecting patient.
- The patient should be in the 'sniffing the morning air' position as for oral intubation.
  - Good positioning is vital in RSI to optimize chances of intubation.
  - One of the most common causes of difficulty intubating is a bad position.
- It is useful to avoid giving a dose of long-acting muscle relaxant after an RSI using suxamethonium, until the patient is seen to attempt to breathe.
  - This avoids the possibility of missing a case of suxamethonium apnoea.

Double lumen tube insertion

- Double lumen tracheal tubes can be used to isolate one lung from the other.
- Several types exist.
- All have similar design (see Figure 4.18)

Indications

- Absolute
  - Isolation of one lung to prevent contamination from the other
    - Unilateral gross pulmonary infection
    - Unilateral massive pulmonary haemorrhage
  - Ventilation of one lung alone
    - Bronchopleural fistula
    - Tracheobronchial airway disruption
    - Giant unilateral lung cyst
- Relative
  - Surgical exposure
    - Thoracic aortic surgery
    - Pulmonary surgery
    - Thoracoscopy/VATS
    - Oesophageal surgery
    - Transthoracic spinal surgery
  - Independent lung ventilation in intensive care
    - ARDS
    - Unilateral lung pathology

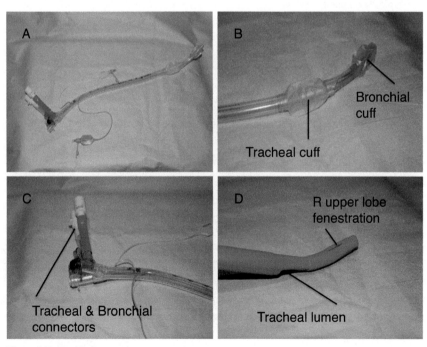

Figure 4.18 Double lumen tube.

Contraindications

- Very few
  - Children under 10–12 years:
    - use a single lumen tube inserted bronchially, or a bronchial blocker.
  - Lesions in a mainstem bronchus would necessitate placement of a tube in the contralateral bronchus.

Complications

- As for oral intubation, in addition to the following.
  - Bulkier tubes make intubation more challenging, and increase the likelihood of laryngeal trauma.
  - Hypoxia may be more likely if intubation takes longer.
  - Malposition is a common problem:
    - especially for right-sided tubes, where occlusion of the right upper-lobe bronchus easily occurs
    - where too long or too short a tube is used
    - due to movement of the tube when positioning patient on the table.
  - Bronchial rupture is rare but serious.

Equipment

- All of the equipment used for intubation as described previously.
- Suction catheters for endobronchial suction.
- Double-lumen tubes are described as 'right' or 'left' sided, according to which main bronchus they are designed to intubate.
- Various sizes of double-lumen tube.
  - Taller or shorter individuals may require larger or smaller tubes than would typically be used.
- An appropriately sized single-lumen tube should be available in case of difficulty placing the double-lumen tube.
- Stylet (if supplied with tube to be used).
- Stethoscope.
- Fibreoptic bronchoscope.
- Clamps.
  - Or other device for occluding either lumen (if supplied with tube to be used).

Sites

- Double-lumen tubes can be placed in right or left main bronchi.

Insertion technique

- This is just one method of insertion and checking position.
- Every centre/anaesthetist will have their own variations on this theme.
- The following method of insertion assumes that there is no risk of contamination from one lung to the other.
- Always ensure that the correct tube (i.e. right or left sided) is being used. Check with the surgical team, and review the history.
- A left-sided tube is used unless it is *absolutely* necessary to use a right-sided one, since the anatomy of the right upper lobe bronchus is unpredictable.

- Insertion
  - The airway should be assessed as for any anaesthetic.
  - A preoperative CXR should be reviewed, paying particular attention to the anatomy of the trachea and main bronchi. If a bronchoscopy has been performed then the results should be reviewed.
  - The stylet that comes packaged with BronchoCath tubes should be inserted into the tube.
  - Check both tracheal and bronchial cuffs.
  - Lubricate both cuffs with water-soluble jelly.
  - Preoxygenate the patient.
  - Perform laryngoscopy.
  - The double-lumen tube should be held so that the tip curves anteriorly.
  - Pass the tube through the pharynx and between the vocal cords.
  - Once the tip is through the cords, rotate the tube through 90 degrees to the left (for a left-sided tube) or right (for a right-sided tube).
  - Advance the tube.
  - Moderate resistance should be encountered as the tube comes to rest in the main bronchus.
- Checking position (Figure 4.19)
  - These tubes are notorious for not being where they should be.
  - Check that the tube is in the trachea.
    - Inflate the tracheal cuff.
    - Ventilate both lumens.
    - Check for E_TCO_2 and bilateral air entry.
  - Clamp the tracheal lumen and open the circuit to air distal to this clamp.
  - Inflate the bronchial cuff slowly while ventilating only the bronchial lumen and listening over the tracheal port. Inflate with just enough air to stop leakage of air from the tracheal port.
    - This will need only 2–3 ml air (if more than 3 ml is needed then the cuff is likely to be partially or completely in the trachea).
  - Next check that the lung with the bronchial lumen can be isolated.
    - Breath sounds and chest movement on the side opposite to the bronchial lumen should cease.
  - Unclamp the tracheal lumen and reconnect the circuit.
    - Both sides of the chest should now ventilate.
  - Next, clamp the bronchial lumen and disconnect the circuit distal to the clamp.
    - Ventilate the tracheal lumen.
    - Breath sounds and chest movement should now be present only on the side opposite to the bronchial cuff.
    - There should be no leaks from the anaesthetic circuit.
  - It is now usual for anaesthetists to confirm the correct position of a double-lumen tube using a fibreoptic bronchoscope. This is more often the case for right-sided tubes where the distal side lumen on the bronchial cuff needs to be placed accurately at the opening of the right upper lobe bronchus.
  - Please note that bronchoscopy does not negate the need for clinical certainty.

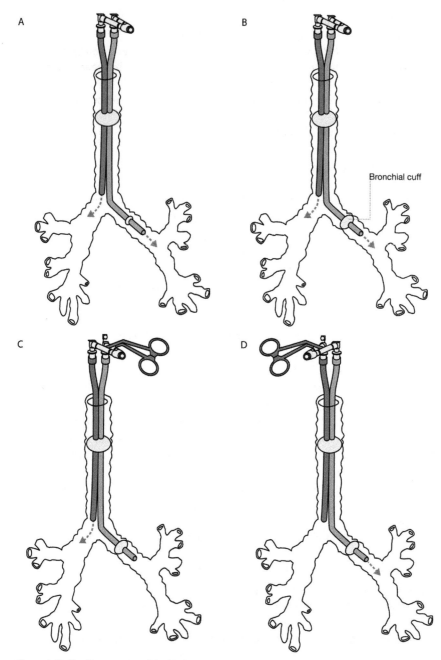

Figure 4.19 Checking position of double lumen tube.

Important points/cautions

- Several types of double-lumen tube are available:
  - Carlens
    - left-sided tube
    - has a 'hook' which sits on the carina and aids placement

- ○ Whites
  - ■ right-sided
  - ■ has a carinal hook and a slit in the tube wall
- ○ Robertshaw
  - ■ right- and left-sided
  - ■ made of rubber
  - ■ used to be reusable; now made in a single-use version
- ○ PVC tubes e.g. BronchoCath
  - ■ right- and left-sided
  - ■ high-volume, low-pressure cuffs
  - ■ bronchial cuff and lumen are blue in colour.
- The most common types in use in the UK are the Robertshaw and the BronchoCath tubes.
- Most modern double-lumen tubes are similar in design to the Robertshaw tubes.
  - ○ Have D-shaped lumina.
  - ○ D-shape allows the largest possible lumen for a given external diameter.
- Tubes are sized in different ways:
  - ○ BronchoCath - 28, 35, 37, 39, 41 F (small to large)
    - ■ the French gauge number refers to the external circumference of the tube in millimetres
    - ■ a 39F double-lumen tube has an external **diameter** of about 13 mm
  - ○ Robertshaw - small, medium and large.
- The lumina of double-lumen tubes are small in comparison to those of single-lumen tubes used. For example, the internal diameter of a 39F double-lumen tube is only 6.0 mm.
- All tubes come in left and right-sided versions.
  - ○ Right-sided tubes have a hole or slit in the wall of the endobronchial section to facilitate ventilation of the right upper lobe.
  - ○ The distance between the right upper lobe bronchus and the carina is only about 2.5 cm in an adult. On the left, the corresponding distance is larger, about 5 cm, so left-sided tubes do not have an eye in the bronchial cuff.
- Checking of tube position with a bronchoscope requires a narrow scope (less than 4 mm diameter).

Tips and advice

- When inserting the tube it may be helpful to turn the patient's head **away from** the side of the main bronchus to be intubated (i.e. to the left when inserting a right-sided tube) once the tube has passed through the cords.
- A rough guide to the depth of tube placement is as follows:
  - ○ for a 170 cm adult, the depth to the corner of the mouth should be 29 cm
  - ○ for each 10 cm change in height, the tube should be inserted further or less far by 1 cm
    - ■ e.g. a 180 cm adult should have a depth of around 30 cm.
- Use the largest double-lumen tube that will pass easily through the cords and not be too close-fitting.
- Incorrect tube placement is the commonest complication. Thorough checking of tube position and adequate ventilation pre- and intraoperatively is mandatory if problems are to be recognized before they cause major complications.

- If there are difficulties in maintaining the airway, a single-lumen tube should be placed, and the double-lumen tube inserted when the patient is stable.
- If the lungs cannot be isolated with a double-lumen tube then alternatives would include bronchoscopic placement of a single-lumen tube in a main bronchus, or use of a bronchial blocker.
- Almost all surgical cases requiring collapse of a lung can proceed with a left-sided double-lumen tube.
- If the patient is moved following intubation (e.g. from supine to lateral position), the position of the tube can easily change. The position of the tube should therefore be checked clinically or bronchoscopically after each change in position.
- Hypoxia can occur if intubation takes longer than anticipated. Be vigilant, and if necessary, reoxygenate the patient before reattempting. Call for help early.
- The bronchial cuff should not be kept inflated for longer than is necessary. It can be deflated when one-lung ventilation is no longer needed.
- Gentle movement of the tube should not result in a leak or a change in ventilation.
  ○ Similarly, higher inflation pressures should not lead to leakage.
- If a double-lumen tube is being used to prevent cross-contamination from one lung to another then the order of cuff inflation and checking should change. The bronchial cuff should be inflated first to isolate the lung and keep it isolated.

Airway devices and 'special' airways

- There exists a multitude of devices to assist with difficult intubations (see DAS guidelines, and Table 4.4).
- Often, careful attention to correct positioning of the patient can resolve difficulties with laryngoscopy and intubation.
- This section focuses only on some of the equipment available for use in these situations.

Indications

- As stated in the DAS guidelines for management of difficult airways (see later section), airway adjuncts and devices should be considered for use early on after discovery of difficulty.
- The choice of device will depend on the situation, the anaesthetist's level of experience and familiarity or lack thereof with the device, and local availability.

Equipment

Table 4.4 Airway devices/special airways

Device/Airway	Description, indications, notable points
Cook airway exchange catheter	• Long, hollow catheter with centimetre markings • Inserted through TT or tracheostomy tube to facilitate change of tubes • Adaptor attached at proximal end (either 15 mm standard or jet ventilator) • Oxygenation possible via catheter • Can also be used in place of a bougie, facilitating oxygenation during difficult intubations
Aintree airway exchange catheter	• Similar in design to Cook catheter • Wider lumen (4.7 mm) to allow for fibreoptic-guided placement of endotracheal or nasotracheal tubes
Cuffed oropharyngeal airway (COPA)	• Consists of a modified Guedel-type airway with an inflatable cuff • Has 15 mm standard connector proximally for attachment to breathing circuit • Can be used during elective anaesthesia with spontaneous or controlled ventilation where there is no aspiration risk
Combitube	• Oesophageal/tracheal airway • Double lumen tube • Introduced blindly into the mouth • Distal tube may enter the trachea or oesophagus • Tracheal channel has open distal end • Oesophageal channel has blind ending and side holes • Two cuffs – one proximal and one distal • No matter where distal tube ends up, ventilation can be achieved • Can be used as a 'rescue' device in difficult intubation
Intubating LMA (ILMA™)	• Modification of LMA • Specially designed LMA inserted first • Specially designed TT passed (blind) through the LMA and into the trachea

Table 4.4 Airway devices/special airways *(Continued)*

Device/Airway	Description, indications, notable points
Lightwand	• A lighted stylet • Introduced through lumen of TT so that lighted end protrudes at distal end • The TT is passed through the mouth in combination with the lightwand • Transillumination allows the tube to be seen passing into the larynx • Backup equipment for direct or fibreoptic intubation should be available
Oesophageal detector	• 50 ml syringe or self-inflating bulb • Applied to the TT connector • Aspiration is attempted • If TT is in oesophagus, aspiration is difficult • 'Free' aspiration indicates tracheal (correct) placement

Video-laryngoscopes

• An increasing number of video-laryngoscopes are available. Examples include:
  ○ Airtraq®
  ○ Glidescope®
  ○ McGrath laryngoscope
• They are all designed to enable the user to visualize the larynx using optical or video technology.
• The devices use optical or video technology to 'place' the viewer's eye at the laryngeal inlet rather than outside the patient's mouth.
• These devices have associated 'learning curves', and can be hard to use initially. **do not** attempt to use a video-laryngoscope unless you have had experience and training in their use, and ensure that a senior anaesthetist is present.

Indications

• Video-laryngoscopes can be used for any intubation, but are usually reserved for situations where a difficult airway is either anticipated, or unexpectedly encountered.
• Certain situations lend themselves to the use of a video-laryngoscope, such as:
  ○ cranio-facial abnormalities
  ○ Mallampati score of 3 or 4 on clinical examination
  ○ previous difficult intubation
  ○ cervical spine immobilisation
  ○ fixed flexion abnormalities of the C-spine
  ○ many more…

Contraindications

• These are the same as for performing conventional laryngoscopy (see earlier section).

Complications

• Failed intubation is still a risk when using a video-laryngoscope.
• The other complications are the same as for conventional laryngoscopy and intubation (see earlier section).

Equipment

• **All** equipment should be checked thoroughly prior to use, to ensure it is in operational order.

- Video-laryngoscope of choice.
  - This will depend on availability locally, and on departmental policies/guidelines.
- Any other equipment recommended or needed for use with the video-laryngoscope.
  - E.g. power supply, monitor, introducer
- An appropriate sized TT that is compatible with the video-laryngoscope being used.
- All other equipment needed is the same as for conventional intubation (see earlier section).

Sites

- Video-laryngoscopes can be used to facilitate oral and nasal intubation.

Insertion technique

- Insertion technique varies depending on the make and model of video-laryngoscope being used.
- The manufacturer's instructions and guidelines should be followed wherever possible.
- Instruction in the use of the video-laryngoscope should be sought prior to use.
- Certain models such as the Glidescope® are similar in appearance to a conventional laryngoscope, whereas others, e.g. Airtraq® are unlike other laryngoscopes and require novel techniques for correct use.
- Some video-laryngoscopes may require a TT to be 'pre-loaded' into a specific channel on the device (Airtraq®), or may require that the TT is inserted as in conventional laryngoscopy with or without an introducer.

Important points/cautions

- As mentioned above, experimentation with airway devices is dangerous and can be lethal. Only use equipment with which you are familiar, and have preferably used in a supervised, clinical situation previously.
- **Ask for help** if you are at all unsure about how to use a video-laryngoscope.
- Practice on mannequins is possible and can be very beneficial prior to use on real patients.
  - Certain manufacturers have training models and mannequins and will usually be happy to arrange for company representatives to run training sessions.
- A video-laryngoscope does not guarantee intubation.
  - A management plan for failure should still exist and a variety of other 'difficult intubation' equipment should be close at hand.
- Maintenance of oxygenation is of paramount importance, and use of video-laryngoscopes can sometimes require a lot of concentration of the part of the operator. Ensure that you do not become distracted. An assistant can be invaluable as they can monitor the patient during intubation attempts.

Tips and advice

- Instruction and practice are invaluable. Try to get hands-on experience with a video-laryngoscope in a safe, supervised environment.
- Ensure that power supplies are fully charged/plugged in and working properly before use. It is also essential to check all connections to any screens or monitors to be used, and that these too are working correctly.

Difficult intubation

- A difficult intubation can be roughly defined as the clinical situation that arises when an appropriately trained anaesthetist experiences difficulty with tracheal intubation.
  - This can be subdivided into difficult **laryngoscopy**, where there is difficulty visualizing the laryngeal inlet with a conventional laryngoscope, and difficult tracheal **intubation**.
  - Difficult intubation is often said to exist when tracheal intubation cannot be performed within three attempts.
- A difficult **airway** can be said to exist when an appropriately trained anaesthetist experiences difficulty with mask ventilation, tracheal intubation or both.
- Difficult airways and intubations can be predicted or unexpected; obviously, the former is preferable!
- Anticipating possible difficulties with intubation or ventilation is a key skill for any practitioner involved with airway management, as is familiarity with algorithms for dealing with these difficulties.
- The following sections follow the guidelines of the Difficult Airway Society (DAS) and some of these guidelines are reproduced with kind permission of DAS.
- Difficulty with intubation and or ventilation can be life-threatening and **every** anaesthetist should be familiar with algorithms or 'drills' which can be followed in case of difficulty.
- The strategy adopted will depend on the clinical situation, and different guidelines exist for managing difficulties in RSIs and in 'normal' elective situations. Guidelines also exist for management of an unanticipated difficult airway.

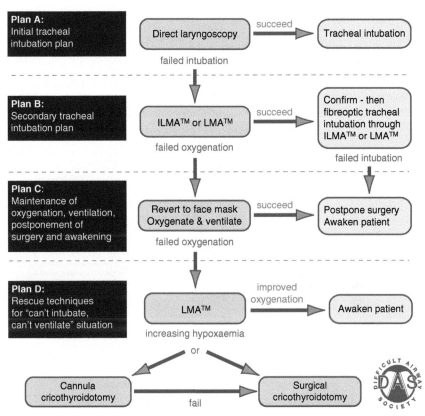

Figure 4.20 Simple composite chart. Difficult Airway Society Guidelines (Reproduced with kind permission of the Difficult Airway Society. For further information visit: http://www.das.uk.com/home).

Failed intubation, increasing hypoxaemia and difficult ventilation in the paralysed anaesthetized patient: Rescue techniques for the 'can't intubate, can't ventilate' situation

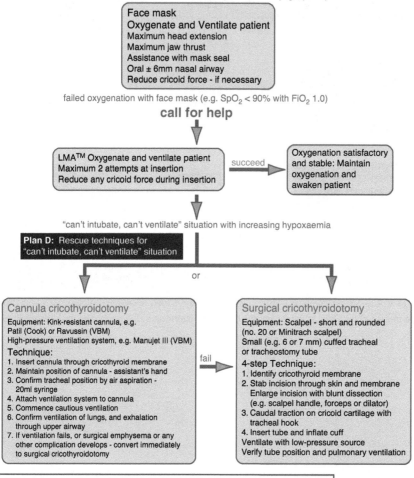

Figure 4.21 Failed intubation, failed ventilation. Difficult Airway Society Guidelines (Reproduced with kind permission of the Difficult Airway Society. For further information visit: http://www.das.uk.com/home).

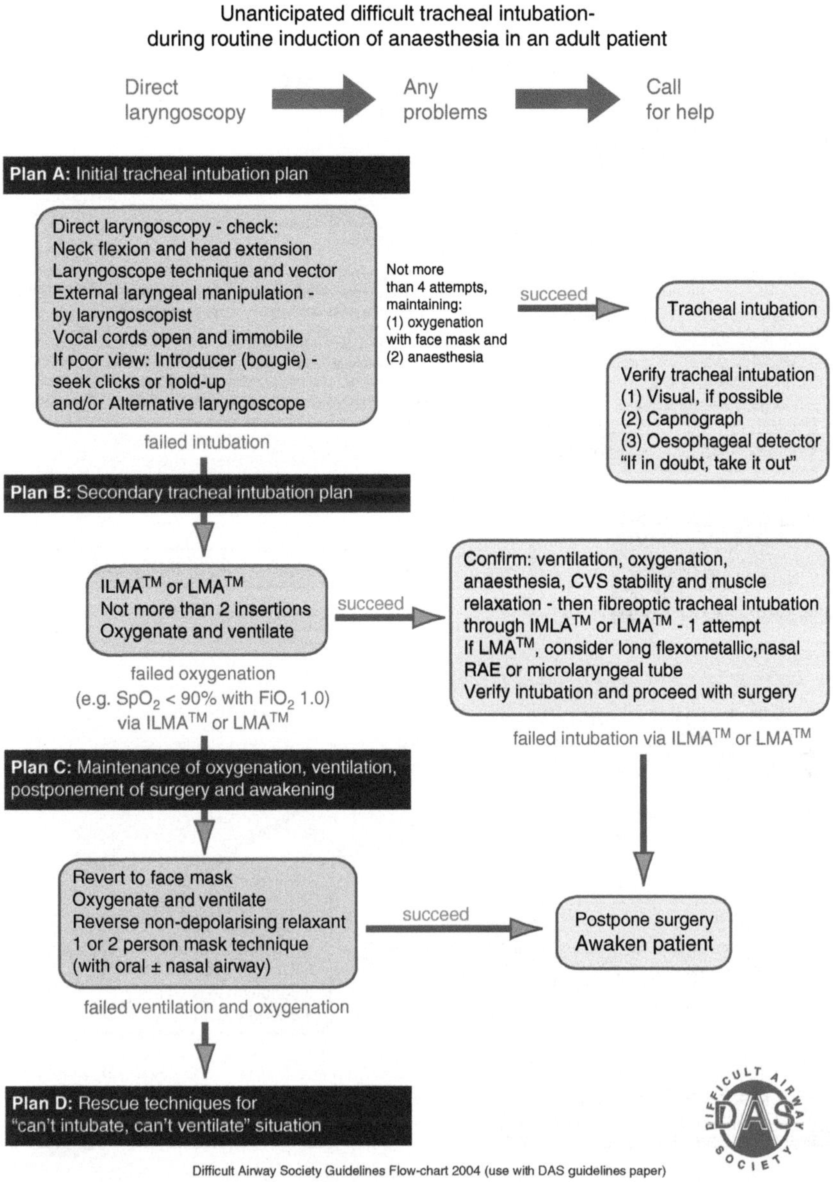

Unanticipated difficult tracheal intubation-
during routine induction of anaesthesia in an adult patient

Direct
laryngoscopy → Any
problems → Call
for help

Plan A: Initial tracheal intubation plan

Direct laryngoscopy - check:
Neck flexion and head extension
Laryngoscope technique and vector
External laryngeal manipulation -
by laryngoscopist
Vocal cords open and immobile
If poor view: Introducer (bougie) -
seek clicks or hold-up
and/or Alternative laryngoscope

Not more
than 4 attempts,
maintaining:
(1) oxygenation
with face mask and
(2) anaesthesia

→ succeed →

Tracheal intubation

Verify tracheal intubation
(1) Visual, if possible
(2) Capnograph
(3) Oesophageal detector
"If in doubt, take it out"

failed intubation

Plan B: Secondary tracheal intubation plan

ILMA™ or LMA™
Not more than 2 insertions
Oxygenate and ventilate

→ succeed →

Confirm: ventilation, oxygenation,
anaesthesia, CVS stability and muscle
relaxation - then fibreoptic tracheal intubation
through IMLA™ or LMA™ - 1 attempt
If LMA™, consider long flexometallic, nasal
RAE or microlaryngeal tube
Verify intubation and proceed with surgery

failed oxygenation
(e.g. SpO$_2$ < 90% with FiO$_2$ 1.0)
via ILMA™ or LMA™

failed intubation via ILMA™ or LMA™

Plan C: Maintenance of oxygenation, ventilation,
postponement of surgery and awakening

Revert to face mask
Oxygenate and ventilate
Reverse non-depolarising relaxant
1 or 2 person mask technique
(with oral ± nasal airway)

→ succeed →

Postpone surgery
Awaken patient

failed ventilation and oxygenation

Plan D: Rescue techniques for
"can't intubate, can't ventilate" situation

DIFFICULT AIRWAY SOCIETY
DAS

Difficult Airway Society Guidelines Flow-chart 2004 (use with DAS guidelines paper)

Figure 4.22 Default strategy for intubation including failed direct laryngoscopy. Difficult Airway Society
Guidelines (Reproduced with kind permission of the Difficult Airway Society. For further information
visit: http://www.das.uk.com/home).

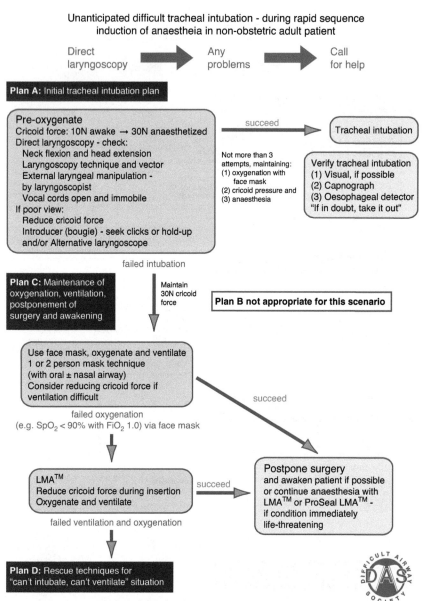

Unanticipated difficult tracheal intubation - during rapid sequence induction of anaestheia in non-obstetric adult patient

Direct laryngoscopy → Any problems → Call for help

Plan A: Initial tracheal intubation plan

Pre-oxygenate
Cricoid force: 10N awake → 30N anaesthetized
Direct laryngoscopy - check:
  Neck flexion and head extension
  Laryngoscopy technique and vector
  External laryngeal manipulation -
  by laryngoscopist
  Vocal cords open and immobile
If poor view:
  Reduce cricoid force
  Introducer (bougie) - seek clicks or hold-up
  and/or Alternative laryngoscope

succeed → Tracheal intubation

Not more than 3 attempts, maintaining:
(1) oxygenation with face mask
(2) cricoid pressure and
(3) anaesthesia

Verify tracheal intubation
(1) Visual, if possible
(2) Capnograph
(3) Oesophageal detector
"If in doubt, take it out"

failed intubation

Plan C: Maintenance of oxygenation, ventilation, postponement of surgery and awakening

Maintain 30N cricoid force

Plan B not appropriate for this scenario

Use face mask, oxygenate and ventilate
1 or 2 person mask technique
(with oral ± nasal airway)
Consider reducing cricoid force if
ventilation difficult

succeed

failed oxygenation
(e.g. $SpO_2 < 90\%$ with FiO_2 1.0) via face mask

LMA™
Reduce cricoid force during insertion
Oxygenate and ventilate

succeed

Postpone surgery
and awaken patient if possible
or continue anaesthesia with
LMA™ or ProSeal LMA™ -
if condition immediately
life-threatening

failed ventilation and oxygenation

Plan D: Rescue techniques for
"can't intubate, can't ventilate" situation

Difficult Airway Society Guidelines Flow-chart 2004 (use with DAS guidelines paper)

Figure 4.23 Failed rapid sequence induction. Difficult Airway Society Guidelines (Reproduced with kind permission of the Difficult Airway Society. For further information visit: http://www.das.uk.com/home).

Retrograde tracheal intubation

- Retrograde tracheal intubation is a useful technique in difficult intubations.
- Often, it is employed where airway lesions are present that would obscure the laryngeal inlet.
- Routinely available anaesthetic equipment can be used, or specially designed kits (e.g. Cook retrograde intubation kit).
- The technique involves the passage of a retrograde guidewire through the cricothyroid membrane in a cephalad direction, and then the 'railroading' of a TT over the wire into the trachea.
- This technique has, to a degree, been superseded by the use of fibreoptic equipment in difficult airway cases.

Indications

- Inability to intubate the trachea using conventional methods.
- Situations where fibreoptic systems are difficult to use, such as:
  - bleeding in the pharynx
  - excessive secretions
  - upper airway neoplasms.

Contraindications

- Unconscious, emergency patients at risk from aspiration of gastric contents.
- Restless, coughing patients.
- Known laryngeal lesions that would make passage of a needle through the cricothyroid membrane dangerous.

Complications

- Failure to intubate the trachea leading to hypoxia.
  - May be due to problems getting the guidewire to pass up through the vocal cords.
- Trauma to the neck, larynx, vocal cords, pharynx, mouth and teeth.
- All of the complications associated with conventional laryngoscopy (see earlier section).
- Bleeding, especially if airway neoplasm is present.
- Laryngospasm.

Equipment

- If a ready-prepared kit is used, most of the following pieces of equipment will be in the kit.
- Cleaning solution (e.g. chlorhexidine)
- 2 ml, 5 ml and 20 ml syringes
- 23G needle for local anaesthetic infiltration
- 1% lidocaine with adrenaline (1:200,000)
- 4% lidocaine
- 18G hollow needle/catheter (e.g. Abbocath), or 16G Tuohy needle
- Guidewire or epidural catheter
- Laryngoscope
- Magill's forceps
- Appropriate size TT
- Water-soluble lubricating jelly

- Artery forceps
- Suction apparatus (switched on and to hand)
- Equipment for ventilation

Sites

- The only site is via the cricothyroid membrane.
- The TT will usually be inserted orally, although nasal intubation is also possible.

Insertion technique

- See Figure 4.24.
- Insertion technique will vary according to whether the patient is awake or anaesthetized.

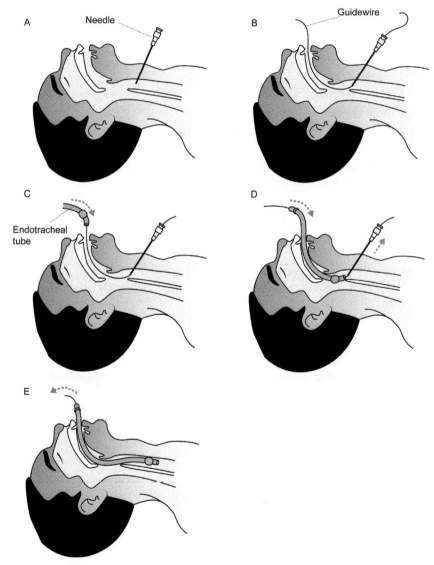

Figure 4.24 Retrograde intubation.

- The patient should be positioned supine with the neck extended.
  - This facilitates access to the trachea.
- Thoroughly clean the neck with antiseptic solution.
- Palpate the thyroid and cricoid cartilages and the cricothyroid membrane between them.
- In an awake patient:
  - draw up 2 ml of 4% lidocaine in a 5 ml syringe
  - infiltrate 1% lidocaine with adrenaline over the cricothyroid membrane with the 23G needle
  - advance the needle through the membrane and confirm that air is aspirated
  - inject 2 ml of 4% lidocaine through the membrane at the end of expiration
  - withdraw the needle **quickly** as the patient will cough
  - these steps are not necessary in the anaesthetized patient.
- Use either the 18G Abbocath or the 16G Tuohy needle to puncture the cricothyroid membrane. If using an Abbocath, 'cannulate' the trachea, removing the needle and leaving the cannula in situ.
  - Have a syringe attached to the needle to aspirate air and confirm the airway has been accessed.
  - The Abbocath should be directed cephalad, or if a Tuohy needle is used, the bevel should point towards the head.
- The guidewire or epidural catheter should be passed through the needle or Abbocath.
- In an awake patient:
  - the guidewire/catheter can be retrieved from the pharynx
  - this may be difficult, especially if the patient has restricted mouth opening.
- In an anaesthetized patient:
  - laryngoscopy should be performed
  - the guidewire will hopefully be seen in the mouth/pharynx and can be retrieved with Magill's forceps.
- Once the wire has been retrieved, an adequate length should be brought out of the mouth.
  - Secure this portion of the wire with artery forceps.
  - The distal end of the wire (protruding from the neck) should also be firmly secured (either by an assistant or with forceps).
  - The TT can then be placed over the wire protruding from the mouth, and the end of the wire held tightly.
  - The TT is then railroaded over the taut wire and into the trachea.
  - Once the TT is in the trachea, the wire is pulled back through the ETT.
  - The TT is then advanced into the correct position.
- The position of the TT should be verified by the usual means.
  - Clinical examination, E_TCO_2 etc.
- In awake patients, anaesthesia can then be induced.
- If nasal intubation is required:
  - a catheter (NG tube or suction catheter) is passed through the nose and retrieved from the mouth
    - the catheter should then be cut so that a short length protrudes from both the nose and the mouth

○ the guidewire from the trachea is passed to the mouth as described above

○ the guidewire is then passed into the catheter leading up to the nose

○ the guidewire can be retrieved from the nose and intubation can proceed as detailed above.

Important points/cautions

● Usually this is a simple procedure.

● If the patient has difficult anatomy such as a thick neck, or if there is inflammation, oedema or bleeding in the neck it may be difficult to feel the cartilages of the larynx and therefore difficult to pass a needle through the cricothyroid membrane.

● In the awake patient, coughing or restlessness may make the procedure impossible.

● If the wire fails to pass easily through the needle then the wire must **never** be forced as the needle is most likely in the tracheal wall.

● The guidewire or epidural catheter must be kept reasonably taut in order for a TT to be railroaded over it.

Tips and advice

● If the patient's anatomy makes it difficult to palpate the cricothyroid membrane, then a 23G fine needle should be used to locate it prior to using an Abbocath or Tuohy needle. This is less likely to lead to unnecessary trauma.

● Occasionally the wire may coil in the trachea and will not therefore pass up through the vocal cords.

○ This may be due to local problems such as supraglottic, glottic, or subglottic oedema, or to partial obstruction of the larynx.

○ Patience and manipulation of the wire may lead to success.

○ Force should **never** be used.

● Caution should be exercised when removing the guidewire and advancing the tube.

○ You should ensure that the tube has entered the larynx prior to removing the wire.

References/further reading

Dhara SS (2009). Retrograde tracheal intubation. *Anaesthesia*, 64 p. 1094–1104.

Emergency airway access

- Having to gain access to the airway in a dire emergency is thankfully a rare occurrence in anaesthetic practice. However, **all** anaesthetists and intensive care physicians should be aware of the following techniques as they can be life-saving.
- Both of the techniques described should be quick and easy to perform, although in an emergency situation even the simplest of tasks can become exceedingly difficult.
- Emergency access to the trachea via the cricothyroid membrane is preferable to surgical tracheostomy as it is less hazardous, usually faster and less complex.
- These techniques appear in the Difficult Airway Society's algorithms (see section on the difficult airway) as 'rescue' techniques in a 'can't intubate, can't ventilate' situation.

Cricothyroidotomy

- This can be performed in the following two ways:
  - Needle cricothyroidotomy
  - Surgical cricothyroidotomy

Indications

- 'Can't intubate, can't ventilate' situation
- Severe anatomical abnormality (e.g. ankylosing spondylitis) making intubation via the larynx impossible
- Maxillofacial or laryngeal trauma
- Laryngeal foreign body that cannot be removed expeditiously
- Upper airway swelling
  - Post-extubation oedema
  - Infections
  - Allergic/immunologic reactions
  - Airway burns

Contraindications

- Absolute:
  - when the airway can be maintained with non-invasive measures
  - in cases where laryngeal, cricoid or tracheal injury makes oxygenation and ventilation via cricothyroidotomy impossible. e.g.:
    - tracheal rupture
    - laryngeal fracture.

Complications

- Failure to access the airway
- Inability to achieve adequate ventilation/oxygenation
- Creation of a 'false passage' resulting in insufflation of oxygen into the para-tracheal tissues
  - Surgical emphysema
  - Pneumomediastinum
- Bleeding
- Air embolism
- Airway barotrauma
  - Pneumothorax

- 'Kinking' of the cannula resulting in difficulty insufflating oxygen
- Hypercapnia
  - Expiration is passive, and may be impeded if the upper airway is obstructed
- Laryngeal trauma
- Subglottic stenosis (late complication)

Equipment
Needle cricothyroidotomy

- This can be performed using a specially designed kit, specially designed cannula or a large-bore IV cannula.
- Several specially designed kits exist, such as:
  - VBM Quicktrach I and II (Ravussin cannula)
  - Cook 'Melker' cricothyroidotomy sets
  - these use a variety of cannula sizes and types
    - some have 15 mm connectors compatible with anaesthetic circuits
  - in an emergency situation, with no access to the above kits, a 14G or 16G cannula can be used, and this is the technique that is described here.
- Equipment necessary for needle cricothyroidotomy:
  - 14G or 16G cannula
  - 5 ml or 10 ml syringe, half-filled with saline
  - antiseptic cleaning solution (if readily available)
  - an injector ventilator (e.g. Sanders injector); if not available then **one** of the following will be needed:
    - a length of oxygen tubing plus a three-way tap or a Y connector
      - if neither three-way tap or Y connector are available then a scalpel can be used to cut a hole in the side of the oxygen tubing (**take care**)
    - a 3 mm/15 mm adaptor from a paediatric TT tube
    - a 7 mm/15 mm adaptor from a TT along with the barrel from a 2 ml syringe
  - High pressure oxygen source.

Surgical cricothyroidotomy

- As with needle cricothyroidotomy, this can be performed using a ready made kit specially designed for this procedure.
  - Several kits are available.
  - Most contain tubes designed specifically for this purpose, and many of these are cuffed.
- The following is a list of the equipment one needs to perform a surgical cricothyroidotomy in the absence of a specially designed kit.
  - Antiseptic solution
  - 5 ml and 10 ml syringes with needles
  - 1–2% lidocaine with 1:200,000 adrenaline
  - Sterile drapes
- All of the above are only used **if time allows**. In an emergency with a hypoxic patient then only the following is needed:
  - Scalpel
    - Disposable plastic with a handle, or:
    - Scalpel handle and number 10 blade

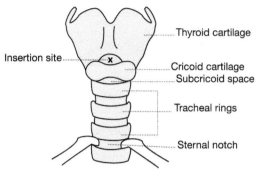

Figure 4.25 Cricothyroidotomy insertion site.

- ○ Artery forceps
- ○ Retractor
    - ■ 'Hook' type retractor
- ○ Lubricating jelly
- ○ 6.0–7.0 mm tracheostomy tube or 6.0–7.0 mm TT (both should be cuffed)
- ○ An appropriate anaesthetic breathing circuit or other means of ventilating
- ○ Suction catheters and functioning suction apparatus
- ○ 20 ml syringe to inflate TT cuff
- ○ Ties or sutures to secure the chosen tube

Sites
- Through the avascular cricothyroid membrane. See Figures. 4.25 and 4.26.
    - ○ This runs from the thyroid cartilage superiorly, to the cricoid cartilage inferiorly.

Insertion technique
Needle cricothyroidotomy
- **Ensure senior help is on the way**.
- Ensure full monitoring is in place.
- Place the patient in the supine position. Extend the neck if possible.

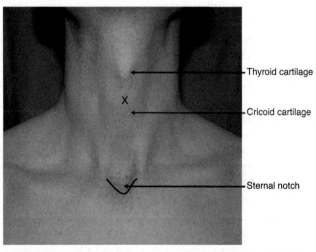

Figure 4.26 Surface anatomy of neck for cricothyroidotomy. X marks the insertion site.

- Palpate the cricothyroid membrane, in the midline, between the thyroid and cricoid cartilages.
- Clean the area with antiseptic solution – if time.
  - In an emergency situation there may not be time to wait for cleaning to occur.
- Attach a 14G cannula to a 5 ml or 10 ml syringe half filled with saline.
- Puncture the skin in the midline, directly over the cricothyroid membrane.
  - Direct the needle at a 45-degree angle caudally.
- Carefully insert the needle through the lower half of the membrane, aspirating as the needle is advanced.
  - Aspiration of air confirms entry into the trachea.
- Withdraw the needle whilst carefully advancing the cannula into the trachea.
  - Take care to avoid the posterior tracheal wall and to avoid kinking of the cannula.
- Attach an oxygen supply.
  - There are many ways of achieving this:
    - if an injector ventilator (e.g. Sanders injector or Manujet) or jet ventilator is immediately available, then it should be used
      - the injector or jet ventilator is attached to the cannula
      - cautious ventilation is commenced, with the driving pressure steadily increased until the chest wall rises
      - if **any** evidence of surgical emphysema occurs, then stop ventilating and proceed to a surgical cricothyroidotomy.
    - A 3.0 mm/15 mm paediatric TT adaptor will fit into the hub of the cannula, and this can then be connected to a standard anaesthetic circuit.
    - A 7.0 mm/15 mm TT adaptor can be inserted into the barrel of a 2ml syringe, and then the syringe attached to the hub of the cannula. This can again be connected to a standard circuit.
    - A 10 ml syringe can be attached to the hub of the cannula, and a cuffed TT can be inserted into the barrel of the syringe, the cuff inflated and the TT attached to a standard circuit.
    - A length of oxygen tubing can be attached directly onto the hub of the cannula. A hole can then be cut in the sidewall of the tubing. This hole is then occluded manually to allow insufflation of oxygen.
      - The oxygen flow rate should be set at 15 L/min.
      - The hole is occluded for 1 second, and then left patent for 4 to 5 seconds. This gives a ventilatory rate of around 10–12 breaths/minute. Alternative set-ups include the use of a Y connector or a three-way tap inserted between the tubing and the cannula. These can then be used to control the flow of oxygen into the trachea.
      - Observe the chest and auscultate, to confirm ventilation.
      - Using this method, expiration is passive and occurs via the upper airway. In cases of partial or complete upper airway obstruction, I:E ratios of 1:8–1:10 (ventilatory rate of 5–6 breaths per minute) should be used. This gives more time for expiration to occur.
- Ensure the patient is being ventilated and that oxygenation is maintained.
  - Monitor saturations and blood gases.
- Secure the cannula in place.
- Seek ENT and senior anaesthetic help with regard to further management.

- **Surgical cricothyroidotomy**
- **Ensure senior help is on the way**.
- Ensure the patient is fully monitored.
- Place the patient in the supine position with the neck extended.
- Identify the cricothyroid membrane in the midline.
- Clean the skin over the cricothyroid membrane and, in an awake patient, consider infiltration with local anaesthetic, only if there is time.
- Make a 'stab' incision through skin and membrane using a scalpel.
  - Enlarge incision with blunt dissection, using forceps or dilator, or inserting the handle of the scalpel into the incision.
- Caudal traction on cricoid cartilage with tracheal hook may be useful at this stage.
- Insert a size 6.0 or 7.0 cuffed tracheostomy tube or TT into the trachea.
- Inflate the cuff and connect to an appropriate circuit.
- Ventilate with low-pressure source.
- Verify tube position and ventilation.
  - Inspection
  - Auscultation
  - Capnography
- Secure the tube in place using ties, tape or sutures.
- Seek ENT and senior anaesthetic help with regard to further management.

Important points/cautions and tips/advice

- With needle cricothyroidotomy, if too vertical an approach is made to the trachea then there is a danger that the inserted cannula may kink and obstruct, making ventilation impossible.
  - This can be avoided by using an angled (caudally) approach or by using a kink-resistant cricothyroidotomy cannula if available.
- In an emergency with an obstructed airway, there may be gross distortion of the anatomy together with engorged neck veins. Coupled with haemorrhage secondary to the procedure, these make the technique difficult to perform.
  - In these situations, the midpoint of the mandible can be palpated and a finger run down the neck to the hyoid bone. This will give an idea of the tracheal position.
- Although these techniques may be life saving, they can be difficult to perform in a stressful, emergency situation. It is therefore vital that all anaesthetists familiarize themselves with the techniques, and if possible practise them on mannequins.
- Haemorrhage on incision is not uncommon when performing a surgical cricothyroidotomy, and functioning suction equipment should be readily available.
- With needle cricothyroidotomy expiration is passive and takes place through the upper airways. It is important to ensure that the upper airways remain unobstructed for this to occur.
- When using low pressure ventilation after larger bore cannulae or endotracheal/tracheostomy tubes have been inserted into the trachea, gases can pass into the upper airway and mouth rather than to the lungs if a cuff is not present on the cannula or tube.
  - Therefore, cuffed tubes should always be used.
  - If a cannula without a cuff is used, then the nose and mouth may need to be held closed by an assistant to allow ventilation to take place.

- Needle and cannula placement in the subcutaneous or paratracheal tissues can lead to disastrous complications.
  - Ensure correct placement of the cannula before using high pressure oxygen ventilation.
  - If there is any suspicion that the cannula is misplaced then cease ventilation and start again.
- A needle cricothyroidotomy can be 'improved' by passing a guidewire into the trachea (through the cannula) and then dilating the stoma and passing a tracheostomy or endotracheal tube into the trachea.
- With both techniques, care should be taken not to pierce the posterior tracheal wall.
- Both of these techniques are for use in emergencies, and are short-term airways. Expert advice from senior anaesthetists and ENT surgeons should be sought as soon as possible in order to create a longer-term airway.

Fibreoptic intubation

- The ready availability of flexible fibreoptic bronchoscopes has revolutionized the management of the patient with a difficult airway.
- Bronchoscopes designed for intubation are usually of a smaller diameter (4 mm or less) than diagnostic scopes used commonly by respiratory physicians.
- The equipment used is expensive and **very fragile**.
  - Care must be taken when using a fibreoptic scope as they are easily damaged in clinical use.
- Fibreoptic scopes may be used in an anticipated difficult airway, or as an emergency aid when unexpected problems arise.
- A fibreoptic intubation may be done in both awake and anaesthetized patients.
- The larynx is innervated by branches of the vagus nerve, the superior and recurrent laryngeal nerves.
  - Superior laryngeal nerve provides sensory innervation above the false cords.
  - Recurrent laryngeal nerve provides sensory innervation below the vocal cords.
  - Any local anaesthetic technique for an awake fibreoptic intubation must block these nerves.

Indications

- Can be used in any situation where direct, conventional laryngoscopy is expected to be difficult or impossible. For example:
  - restricted neck movement or C-spine immobilisation
  - limited mouth opening
  - craniofacial deformities and abnormalities
  - tumour, oedema or haematoma affecting the airway
  - dental abnormalities:
    - overriding front teeth
    - dental abscess.
- Often employed in situations where extension of the neck is to be avoided:
  - C-spine injuries
  - chronic cervical spine abnormalities, such as those that exist in rheumatoid arthritis and ankylosing spondylitis.

Contraindications

- When a definitive airway is needed urgently.
  - Even in the hands of the most skilled practitioners, fibreoptic intubation is time-consuming.
- It is relatively contraindicated where the airway is compromised by excessive bleeding or foreign material, as a good view will be impossible to achieve.

Complications

- In addition to those complications associated with any intubation.
  - Failure to intubate – especially when performed by the inexperienced anaesthetist.
  - Excessive secretions can make it difficult to obtain a good view and can make the procedure hazardous.
  - Hypoxia can occur commonly.
    - Patients often receive sedation.

- ■ The airway may be compromised by laryngospasm or bronchospasm.
- ■ The patient may have a compromised airway to begin with.
  - ○ Local anaesthetic toxicity.
    - ■ Anaesthetizing the airway in the awake patient may require large doses of local anaesthetic.
  - ○ Bleeding.
    - ■ Especially with nasal intubation.
    - ■ This may be profuse.

Equipment

- ● As for all airway procedures, the equipment to be used should be checked thoroughly prior to use.
- ● With fibreoptic intubation it is imperative to check that a power source and light source are both available and working.
- ● Suction should be available, working and ready to attach to the bronchoscope if needed.
- ● The flexible bronchoscope is composed of:
  - ○ insulated glass fibres
  - ○ a light guide cable
  - ○ a working channel for suction oxygen insufflation or local anaesthetic injection.
- ● The bronchoscope has a flexible tip which is controlled with a lever.
  - ○ Movement of the tip in the antero-posterior plane is achieved with the lever.
  - ○ Movement laterally is achieved by rotating the whole scope (see section on bronchoscopy).
- ● The following is a list of the minimum equipment needed to perform a fibreoptic intubation in an anaesthetized patient. This list does **not** therefore include equipment needed to anaesthetize the airway for an awake fibreoptic intubation (see later in this section).
  - ○ Flexible, fibreoptic bronchoscope (external diameter < 5 mm)
  - ○ Working light source (compatible with bronchoscope to be used)
  - ○ Working monitor (if required)
  - ○ Oxygen supply
  - ○ Suction apparatus
  - ○ Nasopharyngeal airways (5, 6, 7, and 8 mm internal diameter)
  - ○ Tracheal tubes (reinforced for nasal intubation)
    - ■ Size 6–6.5 for nasal intubation
    - ■ Size 7–9 for oral intubation
  - ○ Xylometazoline 0.1% (Otrivine®) or phenylephrine 1% nasal spray
  - ○ Mucosal atomisation device (MAD) if available
    - ■ This increases the 'spread' and effect of solutions sprayed into the nostrils
  - ○ If performing an intubation via the oral route then a Berman airway may be useful
    - ■ This allows passage of the bronchoscope through a central channel, and can then be pulled apart for removal prior to TT insertion
  - ○ Small pot containing warm water
- ● As mentioned earlier, there are several methods available for anaesthetizing the airway prior to performing an **awake** fibreoptic intubation. The following list of

equipment is what is required for **one** of these methods, which is preferred by the authors. This is in addition to the equipment listed above.

- Nasal sponge for oxygen administration
- Glycopyrrolate 3 mcg/kg (IV)
- Epidural catheter with the distal end/tip cut off
- Nebulizer apparatus
- 4% lidocaine
- 10% lidocaine spray
- Up to 9 x 2 ml syringes (see later)
- Sterile saline ampoules
- Water-soluble lubricating jelly
- Remifentanil infusion (optional)

Sites

- Fibreoptic intubation can be performed via the nasal or oral route

Insertion technique

See Figure 4.27.

In an anaesthetized patient

- Prepare and check all equipment.
- Connect the bronchoscope to the light source and monitor (if in use).
- The patient should be kept spontaneously ventilating if possible.
- Anaesthesia can be maintained with total intravenous anaesthesia (TIVA) – usually propofol +/− remifentanil.
- Keep the patient on 100% oxygen.
  - Ensure they are well preoxygenated and deeply anaesthetized.
- Load an appropriately sized TT (see above) onto the bronchoscope.
  - This may be secured with tape to keep it in place if needed.
- Pass the cut epidural catheter through the working channel of the scope until the tip just protrudes from the end of the scope.
- Insert the bronchoscope/TT combination via the nose or the mouth.
  - If using the oral route then a Berman airway is useful to direct the scope towards the larynx.
- Have an assistant observe the patient monitor.
  - Watch especially for desaturation and arrhythmias.
- Advance the bronchoscope through the nose or mouth.
- If any obstruction is seen in the nose then it may be useful to try the contralateral nostril.
- The bronchoscope should be advanced through the pharynx until the epiglottis is seen (see Figure 4.28).
- The tip of the scope is then manoeuvred beyond the epiglottis and through the vocal cords.
- The tracheal cartilage rings should be seen, with the carina in the distance.
- Once the scope lies in the trachea, advance the TT over the scope.
  - This may be difficult! Rotation of the TT may aid its passage through the laryngeal inlet.

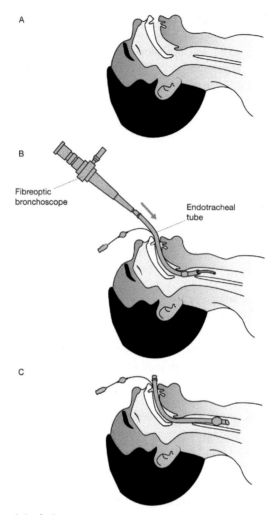

Figure 4.27 Fibreoptic intubation.

- Observe the tip of the TT as the bronchoscope is withdrawn to ensure correct placement.
- Connect the TT to the breathing circuit and confirm correct TT placement.

Anaesthetizing the airway in an awake patient

As mentioned earlier, this is one technique favoured by the author. There are several others.

- Prepare and check all equipment.
- Fully inform and gain consent from the patient.
- Explain the reasons for intubating the patient whilst they are awake.
- The patient may be in the supine or sitting position.
  - The operator may stand behind the patient (head end) or at the side of the bed.
- Find out the patient's body weight and calculate the maximum dose of lidocaine for the patient.
  - Maximum dosage is 9 mg/kg **for this technique only**.

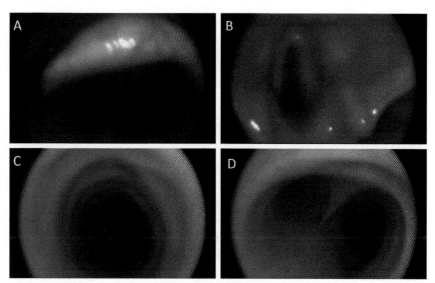

Figure 4.28 Views during fibreoptic intubation. a. Epiglottis b. Vocal cords c. Trachea d. Carina.

- Gain IV access and start infusing crystalloid.
- Give 3 mcg/kg glycopyrrolate IV (max. 200 mcg) to the patient, and spray 1ml 0.1% xylometazoline to each nostril via an MAD (see above).
- Set up a nebulizer circuit.
  - Place 4 ml 4% lidocaine in the nebulizer.
  - Attach the nebulizer to an oxygen supply.
  - Place the mask over the patient's nose and mouth, seal the holes with tape, and tape the edges of the mask to the patient's face.
  - Start the nebulizer with an oxygen flow rate of 5–6 L/min.
- While the nebulizer is running, prepare more local anaesthetic:
  - Each of the 2 ml syringes prepared as follows contains 40 mg of lidocaine
    - Take nine 2 ml syringes.
    - Draw up 1 ml of 4% lidocaine into each.
    - Draw up 1 ml of air into each.
- Once the nebulizer has finished, remove the mask.
- If sedation is being used, then it should be given now.
  - A low-dose remifentanil infusion works well for anxious patients.
  - Usually given at rate of 0.1–0.15 mcg/kg/min.
  - Alternatives include small doses of midazolam or fentanyl.
  - **Beware** the risk of apnoea with sedation, which may be problematic in patients with a difficult airway.
- Identify the most patent nostril and spray 4 sprays of 10% lidocaine into it (40 mg).
- Ask the patient to open their mouth wide and protrude their tongue.
  - Spray 2 sprays of 10% lidocaine to each side of the throat (40 mg).
- Administer supplementary oxygen via a nasal sponge (2–4 L/min).
- Insert the cut epidural catheter through the working channel of the bronchoscope until the end just protrudes from the tip of the scope.
- When the patient is settled, perform the bronchoscopy as described above.

- Further local anaesthesia is achieved as follows.
  - Attach the injection port to the proximal end of the epidural catheter and attach one of the 2 ml syringes with lidocaine/air inside.
  - As the intubation progresses (see above) sprays of local anaesthetic from the 2 ml syringes should be directed (via the epidural catheter) onto:
    - epiglottis
    - vocal cords
    - tracheal mucosa.
  - This will make the patient cough.
  - Ensure that lidocaine sprays are only given **up to** the calculated maximum dose for that patient (9 mg/kg for this technique).
- If all of the lidocaine listed above is used then the total dose will be 600 mg
- In patients of lower body weight the quantity used must be reduced.
- If the oral route is being used in an awake patient, then the same technique can be used, omitting the lidocaine spray and xylometazoline to the nose.

Important points/cautions

- The operator will be focussing on the intubation and the view from the bronchoscope.
  - It is therefore essential that an assistant is present to assist with maintaining anaesthesia or sedation, and with monitoring the patient's condition.
  - Hypoxia can develop during fibreoptic intubations and this should lead to removal of the scope and reoxygenation via bag/mask prior to further intubation attempts.
  - **Full** anaesthetic monitoring and secure IV access should be in place.
- Bleeding from the nose will obscure the view from the scope and make intubation incredibly difficult.
  - Prepare the nose **thoroughly** with xylomatazoline (or an alternative vasoconstrictor) prior to starting.
  - If profuse bleeding does occur, then suction should be attached to the bronchoscope and the intubation may be deferred.
- This technique is not always successful, and the operator should be aware of the limitations of fibreoptic intubation.
  - If intubation is difficult, call for help early and cease attempts when it is obviously failing.

Tips and advice

- A well-informed, fully consenting patient will make the procedure much easier when performed awake.
  - Ensure as much time as needed is spent explaining the procedure to the patient prior to starting.
  - In addition, **low dose** sedation can be incredibly useful in anxious patients.
- There are many ways to skin a cat, and there are also many ways to perform an awake fibreoptic intubation!
  - This is a technique which is learned through 'hands-on' experience in the presence of an experienced supervisor, and this will obviously influence the technique with which one becomes familiar.
- If you are of smaller stature (as one of the authors is) then standing on a raised platform/step will make the procedure much easier to perform, especially if the patient is in the sitting position.

- Some operators find it easier to perform the procedure by passing the TT through the nose and into the pharynx (to a distance of 15 cm) before advancing the bronchoscope.
  - If this method is used then the TT should be softened by soaking in warm water for several minutes prior to insertion (this may be of use in any nasal awake intubation).
  - A naso-pharyngeal airway, cut longitudinally along its whole length, can also be used in this way.
    - As it is cut, it can be removed from around the scope once the scope has entered the pharynx.
- Dipping the tip of the bronchoscope in warm water before starting will help to prevent misting.
- If secretions become attached to the tip of the scope, ask the patient to cough and this may clear them.
- If misting does occur, asking the patient to take a deep breath in will help to clear it.
- If possible, oxygen should be insufflated down the suction channel.
  - This will help prevent hypoxia and misting of the scope.
  - In anaesthetized patients hypoxia can be avoided by attaching a catheter mount with a port in it (see earlier) to the TT, or in certain cases jet ventilation can be used via a trans-tracheal catheter through the cricothyroid membrane.
- In oral intubations, a Berman (or similar) airway can be very useful.
  - In awake patients it will prevent them from biting the scope.
  - If the airway is kept central in the mouth by an assistant, it will help to direct the scope tip to the epiglottis and larynx.
- A fibreoptic bronchoscope can also be inserted through a LMA to facilitate intubation.
  - Once the scope is in the trachea, the LMA can be removed and a TT railroaded over the scope.
  - This can be a useful technique in some difficult airway cases.

Percutaneous tracheostomy

- Percutaneous tracheostomy is an established and respected technique in intensive care practice. It is simple and effective in terms of financial cost, timing of intervention and complication rates.

Indications
Specific
- Bypass obstruction of upper respiratory tract
- Prevent/ reduce aspiration from pharynx or GI tract
- Facilitate aspiration of secretions
- Facilitate long term airway management
- Reduce dead-space
- Allow mobilisation

Additional considerations
- Reduce laryngeal trauma from tracheal tubes
- Easier nursing care
- More comfortable for the patient, less sedation and greater mobility
- Long-term airway protection
- Earlier discharge from ITU
- Easier weaning

Contraindications
- Unstable patient
  - If not vital, wait until the patient is stable.
- Difficult anatomy
  - Short or' bull' neck
  - Enlarged thyroid
  - Inability to feel the cartilages
  - Obesity
    - although often the pre-tracheal area is accessible
- Infection at or near the site
- Coagulopathy is a relative contraindication
- Local malignancy
- Immediate airway access
  - Cricothyroidotomy is the first line; however, tracheostomy can be rapid and effective in experienced hands.

Timing
- At present there is little evidence to support the timing of tracheostomy insertion although this is currently under investigation by the TracMan trial (http://tracman. org.uk).

Complications
Early (during placement)
- Hypoxia
  - Airway management during the procedure is of paramount importance. Hypoxia due to failure of ventilation during the procedure must be avoided by having a trained assistant, preferably an anaesthetist, looking after the airway. The cuff of

the TT may be punctured and make ventilation difficult. This is avoided if the anaesthetist withdraws the tube adequately for access.

- Bleeding
  - Minor bleeding, from skin or the muscle layers, usually settles with placement of the tube.
  - The anterior jugular veins lie in parallel anteriorly over the trachea and are often very large and difficult to see. If perforated they may bleed heavily but are easily accessible.
    - Major bleeding will require surgical exploration especially if the anterior jugular veins or thyroid vessels have been damaged.
    - Significant bleeding into the trachea is hazardous as it may result in blood clot obstructing the airway.
- Wrong level and high stoma
- Paratracheal placement
- Pneumothorax
- Tracheal tear and mucosal flap
- Laryngeal nerve damage (Al-Ansari and Hijazi 2006; Yurtseven 2007)
- Bronchoscope damage
  - Enthusiastic use of a bronchoscope to look for the needle on insertion can result in the 'skin' of the bronchoscope being perforated. This is expensive to replace!
  - The person looking after the airway will be distracted if they perform the bronchoscopy.

Intermediate (days)

- Displacement
  - Particularly hazardous as the entry to the trachea is small and deep and so replacement may be difficult or impossible.
- Obstruction
  - From either blood or secretions.
- Secondary haemorrhage
  - Either from infection or from the local erosion of vessels.
- Infection

Late

- Infection
  - Reportedly 10–30% for surgical and 0–4% for percutaneous tracheostomies.
- Haemorrhage
- Obstruction
- Innominate artery rupture
  - Diagnosed by torrential arterial bleeding into the upper airway. Control has been achieved by performing tracheal intubation and aiming to inflate the cuff at a level which will tamponade the bleeding while surgical correction is carried out.
- Subglottic stenosis
  - The reported incidence is about 4%. It may be associated with pre-existing pathology such as laryngeal oedema or in association with any technique that pushes mucosa or ruptured tracheal cartilage into the tracheal lumen.
- Scarring

Equipment

- Anaesthetist with appropriate intravenous analgesia and anaesthesia
- Laryngoscope
- Tracheal tube for replacement if required
- Suction
- Sterile field
  - Surgical procedure tray or specific surgical tracheostomy procedure tray
- Skin preparation solution
- Local anaesthetic with adrenaline (epinephrine)
- Syringes and needles
- Scalpel
- Lubricating jelly
- Tracheal dilator
- Retractors e.g. self retaining or Langenbeck
- Fibreoptic bronchoscope
- Appropriately sized tracheostomy tube and chosen insertion kit
- 10 ml syringe to inflate cuff
- Catheter mount that accepts fibreoptic scope
- Skin sutures

Insertion of a tracheostomy

- There are two techniques commonly used and several others described.
- Ciaglia uses a wide guided, serial dilational technique with individual dilators.
- The single dilator technique uses a tapered dilator.
- Other techniques include:
  - the Griggs technique with a wire guided forceps
  - the Percutwist which uses a screw technique over a wire
  - the Fantoni technique using a retrograde approach
  - a new technique using balloon dilatation to open the track into the trachea.
- These latter techniques will not be described here.

Equipment

Check:

- Personnel
  - This is a two person technique with one trained person doing the procedure while the other looks after the patient's airway.
- Check your equipment before you start.
  - The operator should always acquaint themselves with the kit before they start.
- Monitor ECG and pulse oximetry.
- The patient should be starved appropriately.
- 100% oxygen.

Positioning:

- Patient
  - Some neck extension to allow optimal access is important, but beware overextension.

- Airway personnel
  - Should have easy access to the airway, the airway equipment and a clear view of the monitoring.
  - Fibreoptic scope should be sensibly placed for use.
- Operator
  - Comfortable with correct bed height and easy access to the neck.

Plan:

- What size tracheostomy tube is needed?
- The tracheostomy tube will have an inner tube so its real size is slightly smaller than anticipated. The patient needs the tracheostomy for easy breathing and access for secretions - use an adequate size.
  - Not less than 8.0 mm in an average female and not less than 9.0 mm in a male. **Do not** use the smallest possible as in anaesthesia. It will increase work of breathing, be more likely to suffer partial blockage with secretions, and prevent easy bronchoscopy.

Insertion technique

- This is an aseptic technique.
- Palpate the neck; identify the thyroid cartilage, the cricoid cartilage and the first tracheal ring. If possible identify the space between the first and second tracheal ring (see Figures 4.29 and 4.30).
- Suction the pharynx to clear secretions.
- Infiltrate local anaesthetic over the space between first and second ring. Solutions containing adrenaline (epinephrine) may help reduce the bleeding initially, but may mask bleeding that could become a problem later.
- Pinch the skin at the entry point with forceps and incise the skin onto the forceps.
  - This minimizes the possibility of hitting an anterior jugular vein.
- Insert the needle down between the tracheal rings or if elective blunt dissect to the trachea before placing the needle (see Figure 4.31).
- If the patient is intubated, ask the anaesthetist/assistant to withdraw the tube to the level of the cords, under direct vision, so that the tube is above the insertion point.
- Control of the airway is vital.
- Introduce the cannula/needle between tracheal rings 1 and 2 aiming slightly caudally.
- Aspirate as the needle advances until the needle is in the trachea and air is aspirated.
  - Saline in the syringe makes it easier to identify air aspiration of air.

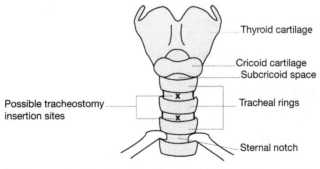

Figure 4.29 Tracheostomy insertion sites. Reproduced with kind permission of Portex, illustrations abridged from Portex originals.

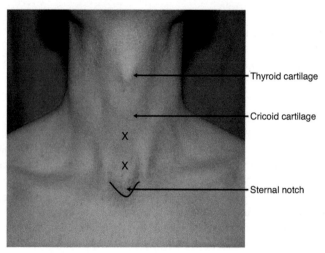

Figure 4.30 Anatomy of anterior neck for tracheostomy. X marks possible insertion sites between tracheal rings. Reproduced with kind permission of Portex, illustrations abridged from Portex originals.

- Remove the needle leaving the cannula in the trachea. Aspirate air again.
- Place the wire through the cannula into the trachea. There should be no resistance.
  - This is when a bronchoscopy will show the wire in the correct position.
- Slide the small firm introducing dilator over the wire, through the soft tissues and into the trachea, feeling a loss of resistance as it passes through the trachea. Remove the dilator ensuring the wire stays in place.
- Place the 'guide' dilator over the wire and advance it until the small cuff is just visible at the skin.

Multiple dilator technique

- Place the smallest dilator over the guide and the wire until it abuts the cuff on the guide.
- Introduce the dilator gently and following the anatomy of the trachea. Usually, this means up to the mark on the dilator, which ensures the tip of the dilator is fully in the trachea.
- Do not hold the wire, as the guide and dilator need to move freely over the wire.
- Repeat with each dilator until one size larger than the tracheostomy to be placed has been inserted.
- Place the tracheostomy tube over the dilator - it will fit snugly.
- Introduce the tracheostomy tube over the wire and dilator guide.
- Remove the wire and dilator guide.
- Connect and check for air entry.
- Perform bronchoscopy and check position.
  - Wash out any blood from the airway.
- Secure the tracheostomy.
  - Stitch the wings to the skin, as this is a dilational procedure and if the tube dislodges it cannot easily be replaced for the first few days.

Single dilator technique

- With wire and dilator guide in place, place the single dilator over the wire and dilator guide until it abuts on the cuff on the guide.

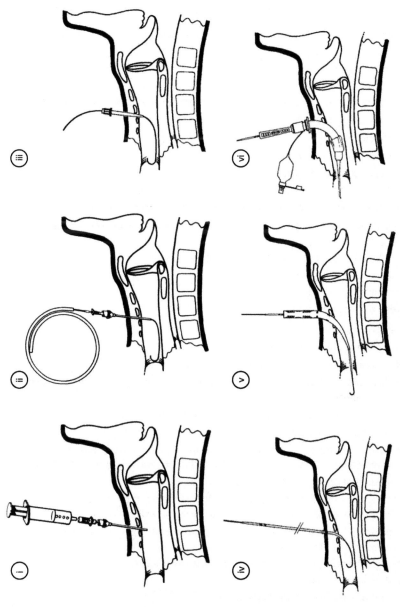

Figure 4.31 Tracheostomy insertion. Reproduced with kind permission of Portex, illustrations abridged from Portex originals.

- Insert the single dilator firmly but gently into the trachea following the tracheal contour up to the mark on the dilator. So that the dilator tip is in the trachea as is the dilator up to its broadest part.
- Do not hold the wire as the guide and dilator need to move freely over the wire.
- Remove the dilator leaving the guide and wire in place.
- Mount the tracheostomy on its introducer and place it over the wire and guide. Push it gently into place.
- Remove the introducer, the guide and the wire leaving the tracheostomy tube in place.
- Inflate the cuff.
- Check its position.
- Perform bronchoscopy to check position. Wash out any blood from the airway.
- Secure the tracheostomy.

Final checks

- Once the tracheostomy is in place:
  - ventilate through the tracheostomy and check air entry to both lungs
    - listen for breath sounds over the lung fields and stomach
    - suction the tracheostomy tube to remove blood and secretions
  - check the site for surgical emphysema which may be an early warning sign
  - secure the tracheostomy
    - stitch the wings to the skin to avoid dislodgement
  - you may wish to perform a fibreoptic bronchoscopy above and below the tracheostomy checking for evidence of trauma
  - keep the kit at the bedside.

Important points/cautions

- Beware the fenestrated tracheostomy.
  - If no inner tube is in situ there will be a massive air leak.
    - A simple, but frequent event that can be disconcerting; corrected with insertion of the inner tube.
- A large mucosal flap can occur and cause obstruction.
  - A mucosal flap may be from the site of entry or posterior wall.
  - If obstruction occurs the priority is to secure the airway. Remove the tracheostomy and reintubate with a TT so that the tube tip is distal to the flap.
    - A surgical opinion is required (ENT).
- If the needle is inserted too far, or if the dilators were forced into the trachea at the wrong angle, a vertical tracheal tear of the posterior wall can occur.
  - It is even possible to perforate the oesophagus. Early signs may include surgical emphysema or airway obstruction.
  - **Surgical emphysema means a complication has taken place and must never be ignored.**
- Later signs of more dramatic tears may include:
  - extending surgical emphysema
  - the nasogastric tube draining air, seen as the 'inflating nasogastric bag' sign, or gaseous distension of the abdomen.
    - Bronchoscopy will show usually a linear posterior tear sometimes into the oesophagus:
      - this may require surgical correction

- temporary solutions include passing an endotracheal tube distal to the tear and allowing spontaneous healing, but this conservative management must be under the auspices of a thoracic surgical team
  - a large tear will require surgical closure.
- In the first 3 days following insertion, before a track has formed, the tracheostomy 'hole' is elastic. If the tube comes out, it will be difficult to replace the tracheostomy, as the hole will close.

Tips and advice
- The needle
  - Can be inserted through the skin but may compress the anterior jugular vein, penetrate it and cause massive bleeding. Although the tracheostomy tube will tamponade the bleeding it is a potential source of ongoing bleeding. This author uses the technique described above to minimize that risk.
- The cannula
  - Once in the trachea do not advance the cannula in further as with a drip; it may kink and make it more difficult to place the wire.
  - Once the wire is in place use a pair of artery forceps alongside the wire to dilate the soft tissues down towards the trachea.
    - In particular stretch the skin incision to be able to accommodate the dilators or dilating forceps and reduce the force required to pass them through the soft tissues.
- The wire
  - Never hold the wire when advancing guides or dilator over the wire. It can kink and thereby allow pressure to be exerted wherever the dilator is pushed.
  - This is how complications such as false passages can occur.
- The bronchoscope
  - In some units the bronchoscope is placed in the trachea to look for the position of entry of the needle.
    - If it is in too far it predisposes to puncture of the scope, as the scope cannot look backwards.
    - It also distracts from the airway management which is vital.
  - It is preferable/sensible to use the bronchoscope to check that the wire is in the trachea once placed.

References/further reading
Ciaglia P, Firsching R, Syniec C (1985). Elective percutaneous dilatational tracheostomy. A new simple bedside procedure; preliminary report. *Chest*, 87 p. 715–9.
Al-Ansari, M. A. and M. H. Hijazi (2006). "Clinical review: percutaneous dilatational tracheostomy." *Critical Care*, 10 p. 202.
Sviri, S., P. V. van Heerden, et al. (2004). "Percutaneous tracheostomy--long-term outlook, a review." *Critical Care Resuscitation*, 6 p. 280–4.
Yurtseven, N., B. Aydemir, et al. (2007). "PercuTwist: a new alternative to Griggs and Ciaglia's techniques." *European Journal Anaesthesiology*, 24 p. 492–7.

Changing a tracheostomy
- Tracheostomy tubes need to be changed, although the interval for change depends on the patient.
- The advent of inner tubes that can be changed easily enables the tracheostomy to be kept clean.

Indications

- Routine changes were traditionally performed after every 7 days or so, but with the use of inner tubes that can be changed there are no set times for changing.
- In the first few days following insertion there is no established track.
  - Try to avoid changing the tube.

Contraindications

- No absolute contraindications.

Complications

Immediate

- Failure to exchange tracheostomy or inability to ventilate post insertion.
- Always have equipment available for direct laryngoscopy and intubation using a standard TT in the event of difficulties placing new tracheostomy.

Other

- As discussed for percutaneous tracheostomy insertion.

Equipment

- Anaesthetic and analgesic drugs as appropriate
- Laryngoscope
- Tracheal tube for replacement if required in emergency
- Suction
- Guidewire or bougie for railroading

Technique

- In a ventilated patient this is a two-person technique (one to look after the airway, the other to change the tube).
- Ideally the patient should be nil by mouth.
- Prepare equipment that would be required to intubate the patient.
- Place patient on 100% oxygen.
- Suction the tracheostomy tube and the pharynx.
- Introduce a wire or bougie into the tracheostomy and then remove the old tracheostomy over the wire.
- Feed the new tracheostomy over the wire/bougie as a guide into the trachea.
- Remove the wire/bougie.
- Inflate the cuff and test ventilate.
- Check the patient is being ventilated adequately:
  - auscultation
  - E_TCO_2 measurement.

Important points/cautions

- Anticipate potential problems that might be encountered, and have all the equipment available that might be required in the event that the tracheostomy change does not proceed smoothly.

Bronchoscopy

- There is a very low threshold for performing bronchoscopy in the critically ill, but it frequently results in a period of ventilatory instability.
- It may be very useful in relieving an obstructed bronchus and hence resolving a collapsed lobe or in retrieving material for microbiological analysis or cytology.
- Frequently it fails in its objectives.
- It is essential to have reasonable defined goals for the bronchoscopy to justify the intervention.

Indications

- Technical
  - Difficult Intubation (see earlier section).
    - Elective:
      - needs forward planning and training in fibreoptic intubation.
    - Emergency:
      - may be useful but not with oropharyngeal bleeding or vomiting.
    - In ICU it is in principle possible but in practice the patient will be too sick or too susceptible to regurgitation.
  - To assist during percutaneous tracheostomy.
    - Can check the position of the guidewire and confirm that there is no posterior wall damage.
- Diagnostic
  - Can be used to check for lesions, foreign bodies.
  - Bronchoalveolar lavage (BAL) and microbiological diagnosis.
  - Biopsy and histology.
  - Tracheostomy position checks.
    - If the lumen abuts the tracheal wall this may be seen.
- Therapeutic
  - Clearing blood or secretions.
    - Especially after a percutaneous tracheostomy where any remaining blood clot has the potential to organise and obstruct.
  - Removing plugs and relieving collapse - best performed when obstruction and collapse has been identified on CXR.
  - Lavage of proteinaceous material.
  - Placing tracheal stents.

Contraindications

- Inexperience with the technique
- Relative:
  - patients at risk of severe hypoxia developing during the procedure
  - presence of profuse bleeding or secretions in the airway.

Complications

- Trauma to the naso/oropharynx is common and obstructs the view.
- Failure to locate the cords:
  - if in doubt **do not** persist.
- Oesophageal intubation:
  - the inner wall is smooth, very different from the trachea and there is no carina.

- Introduction of infection:
  - the scope should be clean prior to use and thoroughly sterilized after use.
- In the anaesthetized patient:
  - temporary obstruction of bronchi can cause collapse
  - it is easy to disseminate infection
  - trauma to the bronchial mucosa
  - bronchoalveolar lavage (BAL) may remove surfactant
  - biopsy can result in bleeding and pneumothorax.

Equipment

- **All** equipment to be used should be checked prior to use.
- The equipment used is expensive and **very fragile.**
  - Care must be taken when using a fibreoptic scope as they are easily damaged in clinical use.
- Flexible, fibreoptic bronchoscope (appropriate size for indicated use).
  - Cleaned, sterilized.
  - With an appropriate, working light source and monitor (if used).
- The flexible bronchoscope is composed of:
  - insulated glass fibres
  - a light guide cable
  - a working channel for suction, oxygen insufflation or local anaesthetic injection.
- The bronchoscope has a flexible tip which is controlled with a lever
  - Movement of the tip in the antero-posterior plane is achieved with the lever.
  - Movement laterally is achieved by rotating the whole scope.
- Right angled connector on catheter mount, with port to accept the scope.
- Suction equipment with sputum trap(s).
- Bronchial brushes and biopsy equipment (if indicated).
- Oxygen tubing connected to oxygen supply.
- Pot of warm water to demist the bronchoscope tip.
- An appropriately qualified assistant
  - To monitor the patient's condition and maintain anaesthesia if necessary.
- 20 ml syringes and sterile saline for flushing if needed.

Insertion technique

- Prerequisites
  - Preoxygenate the patient.
  - Ensure there is an adequate indication.
  - In the awake patient, discuss the benefits and complications and ensure that they are aware of what is to be done and have given consent.
  - Be aware the bronchoscope can be a tool for cross infection.
  - Always have an operator and a separate person to look after the airway and oxygenation.
  - Check the assembly of the scope and light.
    - Ensure that the connectors enable the scope to be used safely if it is being performed on a ventilated patient.
  - Check the scope is working properly.
    - Try to read some printed text through the scope.
    - White balance the scope in accordance with the manufacturer's instructions.

○ Dipping the tip of the scope in warm water prior to starting will help to prevent misting.
- In the awake patient, for intubation see earlier section on fibreoptic intubation.
- In the anaesthetized patient
  ○ Position the patient as required:
    ■ supine or head-up as required
    ■ the technique is most easily performed with the patient at 45 degrees head-up, although this may not always be possible.
  ○ Decide how anaesthesia will be maintained (if necessary).
    ■ Intravenous sedation is usual on the intensive care unit.
    ■ A catheter mount with a port will allow the delivery of volatile anaesthetic agents if required.
  ○ Ensure the catheter mount and connections allow easy passage of the scope and that ventilation can be maintained.
    ■ There is usually a diaphragm through which the scope passes (prevents leakage around the scope).
  ○ Ensure there is full monitoring in place and that a competent person is supervising the airway, anaesthetic and patient's condition.
  ○ Attach suction tubing to the suction port of the scope.
    ■ Turn it on!
    ■ **If** the patient is hypoxic:
      • firstly, think − is bronchoscopy necessary and likely to be of benefit (discuss with your seniors)
      • If so, oxygen should be insufflated via tubing on the suction port instead.
  ○ Look through the scope.
    ■ An indented 'marker' will be visible
    ■ This is used to orientate the scope position (i.e. so you know what is up and what is down).
  ○ The operator will usually stand at the patient's head, or at their side
    ■ Obviously, the position of the operator relative to the patient will alter which side of the view corresponds to left and right sided structures.
    ■ Bear this in mind as the procedure progresses.
  ○ Advance the scope gently through the port on the catheter mount.
  ○ As the scope passes through the TT the walls of the tube will be visible initially.
    ■ Following this, the carina and trachea should come into view.
    ■ Identify the carina and orientate yourself as to which main bronchus is left and which right.
    ■ If standing at the patient's head, the left main bronchus will be on the left of the view. If standing at the patient's side, the left main bronchus will be on the right of the view (this is true as long as the scope has not been rotated).
  ○ The relevant anatomy should be borne in mind as the procedure progresses (see Figure 4.32).
    ■ The left main bronchus arises at a more acute angle than the right, so the right is more clearly seen.
    ■ The right main bronchus gives off the right upper lobe bronchus roughly 2.5 cm from the carina.
    ■ The left main bronchus gives off the left upper lobe bronchus arises around 5 cm from the carina.

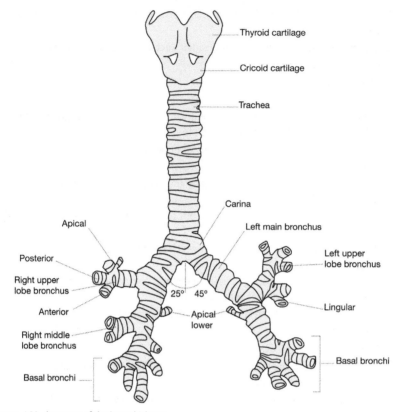

Figure 4.32 Anatomy of the bronchial tree.

- The scope should be directed into one lung first, and then withdrawn to the carina before inspecting the opposite lung.
  - The manner in which the procedure happens will depend on the indication and is often guided by clinical and radiological findings.
- The appropriate biopsies, samples or lavage/suction should be performed.
  - Following any of the above, the airway should be inspected for bleeding as the scope is removed
  - Lavage can be performed by instilling saline down the working channel of the scope and then activating the suction
  - A sputum trap can be used (in the suction circuit) to collect specimens.
- The entire airway should be inspected as the scope is slowly withdrawn.
- After the scope has been withdrawn completely, ensure the patient is ventilated adequately.

Important points/cautions

- If the patient is not very deeply anaesthetized or sedated then coughing may occur on performing bronchoscopy.
  - Muscle relaxation should be considered.
- Ensure you are aware of any anatomical variants or pathology that may make the procedure complicated:
  - e.g. previous airway or lung surgery

- Active infection or airway oedema can make the anatomy difficult to recognize.
  - If the patient is stable, then take time to identify structures such as the carina and lobar bronchi to help orientation.
  - If one becomes 'lost' then gently withdraw the scope to an identifiable anatomical structure before proceeding again.

Tips and advice

- See earlier section on fibreoptic intubation.

Ventilation

- Ventilation is the process by which gases get to the alveoli of the lungs.
- It can be spontaneous or artificial/mechanical.
- There are many modes of artificial/mechanical ventilation available.
- Spontaneous ventilation involves the creation of a negative intrathoracic pressure.
  - Contraction of diaphragm alone or in combination with other muscles leads to negative pressure in thorax, air moves in via the airways.
  - Expiration is usually passive, though may be assisted by thoracic muscles, e.g. in exercise.
- Mechanical ventilation usually involves positive pressure to 'drive' gases into the airways.
  - Negative pressure mechanical ventilation is possible, but not commonly used. Tank/cuirasse ventilation uses negative pressure to mimic normal breathing.
  - The use of positive pressure creates the possibility of damage to the patient's airways.
    - Barotrauma – trauma secondary to high airway pressures.
    - Volutrauma – trauma secondary to high tidal volumes.
- Minute ventilation or minute volume.
  - This is the volume of gas ventilated in one minute.
  - Minute volume (ml/min) = tidal volume (ml) x respiratory rate (breaths/min)
- Alveolar ventilation
  - Volume of gas available to the alveolar membrane per minute.
  - Alveolar ventilation = (tidal volume – dead space) x respiratory rate
  - Dead space is the volume of the inspired gas that is not in effective balance with perfusion.
    - Anatomical deadspace but also good ventilation and poor perfusion.
- Ventilation is a huge topic and several books have been written devoted entirely to it. The following section is therefore a **brief** overview of the basic settings and physiology of mechanical ventilation.
  - It is important to familiarize oneself with the particular ventilator(s) in use in one's institution.
    - If you are **at all unsure**, seek senior help.

Mechanical ventilation

Indications

- The **absolute** indication for starting mechanical ventilation is where the patient is unable to ventilate/breathe for themselves; the indications for intubation/protection of the airway are far more diverse and include airway protection, facilitating ventilation and allowing access to the airway for ventilation, such as with surgery for head and neck (shared airway), or because muscle relaxants necessitate ventilation.
- Obviously any intubated patient may require some form of mechanical ventilation although they clearly can also breathe spontaneously through the tube.
- Some indications for mechanical ventilation are as follows.
  - Ventilatory failure where the motor mechanism of breathing has failed.
  - Respiratory failure where oxygenation is poor, spontaneous ventilation is not sufficient, and where ventilation and gas exchange can be enhanced with positive pressure ventilation.

- ○ Manipulation of blood gases.
  - ■ E.g. in raised ICP where normocapnia is desirable
- ○ In critically ill patients with severe systemic illnesses.
- ○ Respiratory failure:
  - ■ sepsis
  - ■ following cardiac arrest
  - ■ acid–base disturbances
  - ■ when increased oxygen demand cannot be met by spontaneous ventilation.

Settings and modes

This is not intended to be comprehensive but merely to outline the basic principles.

- Modern intensive care ventilators are sophisticated devices.
  - ○ Computer controlled.
  - ○ Multiple ventilatory modes.
  - ○ Inbuilt monitoring and alarm systems.
- Most intensive care practitioners use only a very small number of the available ventilatory modes.
  - ○ Most of the complicated ventilatory modes are used when patients are being weaned from artificial ventilation.
- Sensors are usually present in the ventilator and are therefore distal from the patient.
  - ○ There are almost invariably time delays in the detection of problems.
- Controlled mandatory ventilation (CMV)
  - ○ Simplest form of mechanical ventilation.
  - ○ Patient is ventilated at a preset rate with a preset tidal volume.
    - ■ E.g. 500 ml x 12 breaths per minute
  - ○ Suitable mode for heavily sedated/anaesthetized and/or paralysed patients.
    - ■ I.e. those making **no** respiratory effort.
    - ■ **Not** suitable for patients attempting to take spontaneous breaths or for weaning.
      - • The ventilator may attempt to deliver a breath on top of the patient's spontaneous breath, which is uncomfortable and distressing.
      - • May result in trauma to the airway.
  - ○ Simple set–up guidelines.
    - ■ Check the ventilator has power and gas supplies connected as appropriate.
    - ■ Ensure the patient is sedated and/or paralysed appropriately.
    - ■ Set the following settings prior to connecting the patient to the ventilator (these are only a guide, and the patient's clinical condition, reason for ventilation and blood gases will all affect the chosen settings):
      - • tidal volume (V_T), 7–10 ml/kg body weight
      - • respiratory rate (RR), 8–12 breaths/minute
      - • FiO_2, 0.3–0.6
      - • inspiratory to expiratory ratio (I:E), 1:2–1:3
      - • positive end expiratory pressure (PEEP), 0–5.
    - ■ Connect the ventilator circuit to the catheter mount on the patient's endotracheal tube.
    - ■ Confirm air entry bilaterally.

- Ensure the patient is stable.
- Recheck the blood gases after 10–15 minutes.
  - Does not allow spontaneous breathing activity.
- Synchronized intermittent mandatory ventilation (SIMV)
  - Allows a variable degree of spontaneous respiratory activity.
  - Originally designed to assist weaning.
  - Tidal volume and respiratory rate are preset.
  - Immediately prior to each artificial breath, there is a small window of time during which the ventilator can 'sense' an attempted breath from the patient.
    - If the ventilator senses spontaneous respiratory activity it responds by delivering the mandatory breath early.
    - This avoids breath 'stacking' which leads to high intra–thoracic pressures.
      - Decreases barotrauma and CVS side effects associated with CMV.
- Pressure–controlled ventilation (PCV)
  - Commonly available mode, in theatre and intensive care.
  - Unlike with CMV, in PCV the inspiratory pressure rather than the tidal volume is preset at a desired level.
  - Tidal volume therefore depends on the resistance and compliance of the breathing circuit and the patient's respiratory system.
  - This mode avoids high peak airway pressures, but raises **mean** airway pressure.
  - The achieved tidal volumes must be monitored closely as any change in compliance will cause them to increase or decrease.
- Pressure support or assisted spontaneous breathing (PS or ASB)
  - These modes are primarily used for weaning.
  - As a patient is weaned they will need to do more of the work of ventilation for themselves, but will require some assistance as breathing through a ventilator and circuit is difficult.
  - Pressure support assists the patient who is spontaneously breathing.
    - The ventilator senses a patient's attempt to take a breath.
    - The ventilator then augments the breath with the addition of positive pressure (at a preset level).
      - Reduces the work of breathing.
      - Increases the tidal volume.
  - Pressure support levels of 15–20 cmH_2O are usual initial settings, and this is reduced as the patient recovers.
- Positive end expiratory pressure (PEEP)
  - Intubation and mechanical ventilation both decrease a patient's FRC.
    - This leads to small airways collapse, shunt and worsening gas exchange.
  - PEEP involves the maintenance of airway pressure above atmospheric pressure at the end of expiration.
    - This helps prevent small airways collapse by increasing FRC.
    - Recruits collapsed alveoli.
    - Reduces the work of breathing.
    - Improves oxygenation by reducing shunt.
    - Levels of 5–15 cmH_2O are commonly used.
    - High levels often used in ARDS patients.
  - PEEP is relatively contraindicated in patients with asthma or emphysema.

- Continuous positive airway pressure (CPAP)
  - CPAP is similar to PEEP, but in the spontaneously breathing patient.
  - It can be invasive or noninvasive.
    - Noninvasive CPAP requires the use of a tight−fitting mask.
    - Often used in combination with pressure support in weaning.
  - CPAP has similar effects to PEEP (see above).
  - CPAP can be delivered via continuous, high−flow systems or via a ventilator.
  - CPAP levels of between 5 and 10 cmH$_2$O are commonly used.
  - 'Wall' CPAP is very noisy and can be difficult to humidify.
- Bi−level positive airway pressure (BiPAP)
  - Mode of noninvasive ventilation that is similar to pressure support and CPAP in intubated patients.
  - Involves the use of a tight−fitting mask.
    - Mandates a conscious, cooperative patient.
  - Two levels of pressure are preset.
    - IPAP
      - Inspiratory positive airway pressure (usually 10−25 cmH$_2$0)
    - EPAP
      - Expiratory positive airway pressure (usually 4−15 cmH$_2$0)
  - The BiPAP machine maintains a baseline pressure of at least the EPAP level.
  - When the patient makes respiratory effort, the machine senses this (negative pressure) and supports the breath by adding positive pressure up to the set IPAP level.
  - BiPAP can help to improve oxygenation (as with CPAP), but also helps to increase the elimination of CO$_2$ by increasing alveolar ventilation.
  - BiPAP is indicated in:
    - COPD exacerbations
    - neuromuscular disorders
    - cardiac failure
    - type 2 respiratory failure.
- High−frequency ventilation
  - High−frequency jet ventilation (HFJV)
    - Often used in theatre for head and neck/ENT and thoracic surgical procedures.
    - Rigid bronchoscopy
    - Laryngeal surgery
    - Laser surgery to the airway
    - Can be used via transtracheal or transcricothyroid routes in difficult airways.
    - Involves respiratory rates of 60−150 breaths/minute.
      - Jet of oxygen +/− air directed via small diameter cannula.
      - Either from a jet ventilator machine or from a handheld (Sanders) injector.
      - The driving pressure is set to achieve chest wall movement.
      - Initial settings are usually:
        FiO$_2$ 0.6−1.0
        driving pressure 1.5−3.0 atm
        I:E 1:1

- V_T is around 70–150 ml.
- Expiration is passive.
- Care must be taken to avoid barotrauma.
- Although oxygenation may be maintained, CO_2 is harder to remove.

- High–frequency oscillation (HFO)
  - Uncommon in adult practice.
  - More usually encountered in paediatric intensive care.
  - Involves respiratory rates of 180–3000 breaths/minute.
  - A piston oscillates a diaphragm across the open airway.
    - Leads to a sinusoidal flow pattern.
    - Both inspiration and expiration are active.
    - Mean airway pressure is increased to recruit alveoli and improve oxygenation.
    - CO_2 clearance is achieved by increasing the respiratory rate.

Important points/cautions

- All patients undergoing any form of artificial ventilation should be closely monitored in a suitable environment.
- Ventilatory parameters need to be adjusted often and this will be dictated by the patient's clinical condition and arterial blood gases.
- Positive pressure ventilation has many associated side effects. The most serious are the cardiovascular and respiratory ones.
- CVS side effects:
  - increased intrathoracic pressure impedes venous return and lowers cardiac output
    - trying to prevent high airway pressures will help to avoid the above
  - this phenomenon is compounded by the use of PEEP
  - CPAP and BiPAP can also affect cardiac output in this way.
- RS side effects:
  - positive pressures applied to the airway can lead to trauma
  - barotrauma and volutrauma
    - peak airway pressures should be limited to < 30 cmH$_2$0 wherever possible
    - tidal volumes of 6–8 ml/kg can be used to avoid volutrauma
  - opening of collapsed airways and trauma caused by overdistension of alveoli can lead to cytokine release and cause a systemic inflammatory response (SIRS)
    - repeated opening and closing of small airways can be avoided with the use of PEEP.
- Modern ventilatory strategies, especially in ARDS patients, may focus on improving oxygenation and tolerating raised $PaCO_2$ levels as a side effect.
  - This is so–called 'permissive hypercapnia.'
- Noninvasive ventilation (NIV) has revolutionized the management of respiratory failure, especially in COPD patients.
  - Both CPAP and BiPAP are useful but have limitations.
  - Uncooperative patients will not tolerate a tight–fitting mask.
  - Patients with decreased conscious levels will be at risk of aspiration.
  - The masks can cause pressure sores on the face.

- Departmental protocols should be followed wherever they exist, and these should give clear guidance on when a patient should be intubated if NIV is failing.
- CPAP systems involving the used of 'hoods' applied over the patient's head are sometimes better tolerated than facemask systems.

Chapter 5
Thoracic Procedures

Needle thoracostomy for chest aspiration

Indications

- Decompression of tension pneumothorax.
- Diagnosis, with or without aspiration (removal), of pneumothorax, pleural effusion or haemothorax.

Contraindications

Relative

- Coagulopathy
- Local skin infection overlying insertion site
- Loculated effusions
- Positive pressure ventilation
  - Increased risk of pneumothorax

Complications

- Haemorrhage.
  - Avoid intercostal vessels by introducing the needle above, rather than below, the rib margin (see Figure 5.1).
- Loculated effusions may be difficult to drain.
- Damage to pleura leading to pneumothorax.
  - If there was no pneumothorax the pleura will almost certainly have been punctured by the procedure.
- Infection.
- Pulmonary oedema.
  - Can occur following rapid removal of large volume of pleural fluid with consequent rapid lung re–expansion.
- Tube blockage, particularly with blood, has several effects.
  - May result in pressure or fluid build up in the chest.
  - Misguides as to actual fluid/blood loss.

Aspiration of tension pneumothorax

- Tension pneumothorax is a medical emergency and requires rapid and effective correction as soon as the diagnosis is made (see Figure 5.1).

Equipment

- Antiseptic solution
- 16G or 14G cannula
- Gauze and tape

Sites

- Mid clavicular line, second intercostal space (see Figure 5.2)

Insertion technique

- See Figure 5.3.
- Position patient supine, slight head up position if possible.
- Clean skin.
- Confirm correct side for drainage.
- Insert cannula at 90 degrees to skin over the upper rib margin until a loss of resistance or pop is felt (penetration of parietal pleura).

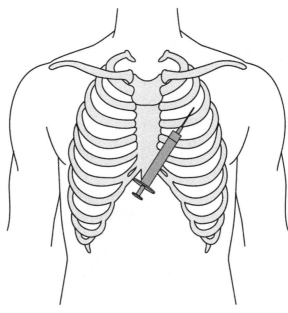

Figure 5.1 Illustration of insertion site for needle thoracostomy.

- Remove needle while advancing cannula.
- An obvious escape of air should be demonstrated with a hissing noise.
- Secure the cannula in place pending insertion of a definitive chest drain.
  - Leave cannula open if on positive pressure ventilation.
  - Close cannula if breathing spontaneously.
- Make arrangements for insertion of surgical chest drain.
  - This should be a large chest drain, as it must provide a low resistance method for air to escape.

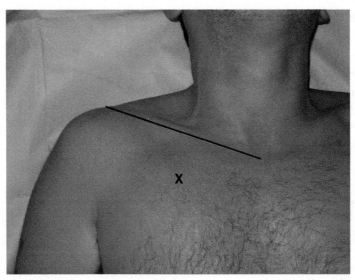

Figure 5.2 Insertion point for needle thoracostomy.

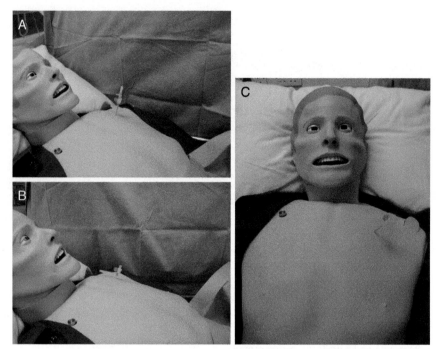

Figure 5.3 Insertion of cannula for needle thoracostomy. Demonstrated on manikin. A and C demonstrate cannula insertion site B: Needle removed, cannula in place.

Important points/cautions
- Ensure the cannula is secured as dislodgement may result in reaccumulation of pneumothorax.

Tips and advice
- Use largest bore cannula available.

Aspiration of pleural effusion/haemothorax

Equipment
- Antiseptic solution
- 18G or 16G cannula
- 1% lidocaine, 5 ml syringe
- 20 ml or 50 ml syringe
- Three-way tap
- Gauze and tape

Sites
- Varies depending on the site of the effusion, especially if loculated.
- Assess with percussion, auscultation, CXR and CT scan (optional).
- In the conscious patient:
  - commonly undertaken via an intercostal space in the mid-scapular line.
- In the unconscious patient:
  - usually performed via chest drain insertion (see later) in the 5th intercostal space and mid-axillary line.
- See Figure 5.4.

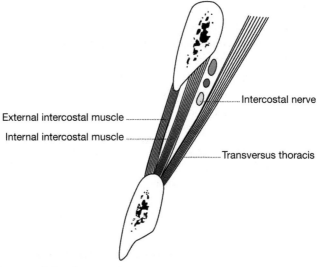

Figure 5.4 Anatomy of rib and intercostal space.

Insertion technique

For the conscious, cooperative patient.

- Have patient adopt a sitting position, leaning forward over a table or with elbows resting on a table (see Figure 5.5).
- Percuss the effusion's upper and lower limits and choose a suitable intercostal space in between these two points.
- Clean the skin overlying the insertion site.
- Drape the skin and ensure that you adhere to an aseptic technique.
- Infiltrate the skin with local anaesthetic.
- Insert a 21G needle (for diagnostic taps) or 16G cannula (for fluid removal).

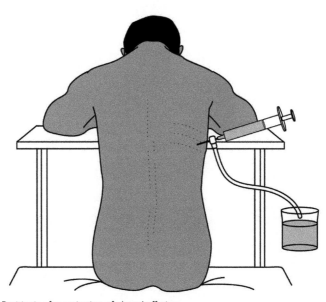

Figure 5.5 Positioning for aspiration of pleural effusion.

- Remove the needle from cannula.
- Attach 50 ml syringe via a three–way tap.
- Aspirate pleural fluid into syringe, turn three–way tap and expel fluid.
  - Avoids possible air entrainment into the pleural space.
- Continue until all fluid aspirated (see cautions below).
- Remove cannula and apply suitable dressing.
- Examine CXR for any pneumothorax.

Important points/cautions

- It is important to map out the effusion to avoid causing damage to the diaphragm at the lower border and the lung at the upper border.
- It is generally advised to remove a maximum of 1 litre of fluid at any one time and to do so slowly.
  - Pulmonary oedema can result if large volumes are removed quickly.

Tips and advice

- Ensue patient in a comfortable position prior to starting procedure to minimize need for movement during procedure.
- When aspirating a pleural effusion using a cannula and a three–way tap, an IV giving set with the drip chamber cut off can be attached to one port of the three–way tap and the other end can be placed in a collecting vessel on the floor. As the fluid is aspirated using a syringe, the three–way tap can be turned to direct the fluid down the giving set and into the collection vessel.
  - This is very useful when large volumes are to be aspirated.

Intercostal drain insertion

- There are two methods of inserting an intercostal chest drain.
- The surgical technique is a procedure carried out under direct vision (i.e. no needles are 'blindly' inserted into the chest wall).
  - Typically the drains inserted are larger than those inserted using the Seldinger technique.
- The Seldinger technique relies on the location of the pleural space with a needle (now often assisted with the use of ultrasound) and the insertion of a guidewire, with subsequent insertion of the drain over the wire.
  - Typically these drains are smaller.
- The choice between the two techniques depends upon local and personal preferences, the fluid being drained, and patient factors.
- The narrower tube has a higher resistance and is more likely to occlude, but is more comfortable and less intrusive for the patient.

Surgical chest drain insertion

Indications
- Pleural effusion
- Pneumothorax (positive pressure ventilation, postoperative, post–traumatic)
- Tension pneumothorax after initial needle relief
- Haemothorax
- Empyema drainage
- Chyle drainage

Contraindications
- Relative
  - Coagulopathy
  - Local infection

Complications
- Misdiagnosis, resulting in pneumothorax.
- Incorrect placement:
  - lying outside parietal pleura resulting in no drainage
    - there will be no 'swing' on the underwater seal but the CXR may appear to show acceptable drain placement
  - under the diaphragm with consequent risk of iatrogenic injury (and failure of chest drainage).
- Organ damage:
  - lung, heart, oesophagus, blood vessels, diaphragm, spleen and liver
  - especially if a trocar is used.
- Haemorrhage, usually from an intercostal artery or vein.
- Infection.
- Drain blockage:
  - especial risk in presence of haemothorax
  - use largest drain practical to prevent blockage in presence of blood.
- Surgical emphysema:
  - air leak through parietal pleura but not through skin

○ this can occur if resistance though drain is higher than that through surrounding tissue i.e. drain blockage.

Equipment

- Antiseptic solution and sterile drapes
- Lidocaine 1–2%
- Chest drain 10–36 Ch
- Scalpel
- Artery forceps
- Blunt forceps
- Skin suture
- Needle holder
- Gauze
- Dressing
- Underwater seal drainage system
- Sterile water to fill seal chamber

Sites

- Anterior approach:
  ○ second intercostal space, mid clavicular line
  ○ lateral to the internal mammary artery
  ○ cosmetically inferior
  ○ potentially anatomically more favourable for drainage of air as near apex of lung.
- Lateral approach (see Figure 5.6).
  ○ more common in anaesthetic/intensive care practice
  ○ mid axillary line, 5th or 6th intercostal space
  ○ adequate for fluid drainage, especially if patient supine
  ○ less overlying muscle
  ○ greater potential for damage to the diaphragm.

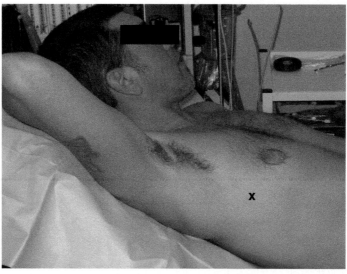

Figure 5.6 Lateral chest drain insertion site.

Insertion technique

- See Figure 5.7.
- Confirm diagnosis; ultrasound can be effectively used as a bedside technique.
  ○ Check position of diaphragm on CXR.
- Position patient (see photo, Figure 5.6).
- Sterile technique.
- Locate 5th or 6th intercostal space, mid–axillary line.

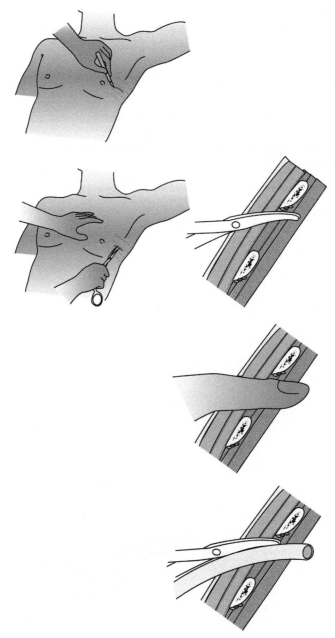

Figure 5.7 Surgical placement of a chest drain.

- Infiltrate local anaesthetic over the insertion site.
- Make incision in skin parallel to the rib over intercostal space, large enough for selected drain to pass through (2–3 cm).
- Avoiding lower margin of rib (where the neurovascular bundle runs), use forceps (large and blunt) for blunt dissection through intercostal muscles down to the pleura.
- Push forceps gently through into the pleural space.
- Introduce a finger into the space and perform a sweep.
  - Confirms pleural space entered.
  - May give information as to the condition of the lung and presence of adhesions.
- Using the forceps, introduce the chest drain.
  - Aim cephalad if draining air.
  - Aim posteriorly if draining fluid.
- Connect the drain to an underwater seal system (or a chest drainage bag).
  - Check the fluid in the tubing 'swings' with ventilation.
- Close each side of the incision around the drain with mattress sutures.
- Place a purse string suture around the incision and wind it several times around the drain before tying it securely (see Figure 5.8).
- Perform CXR to confirm placement (see Figure 5.9)

Important points/cautions

- **Never** use a trocar to place a chest drain.
  - Blind insertion of a trocar can result in serious damage to lung, blood vessels, heart and intra–abdominal organs.
  - Discard any trocar supplied with a drain before insertion.

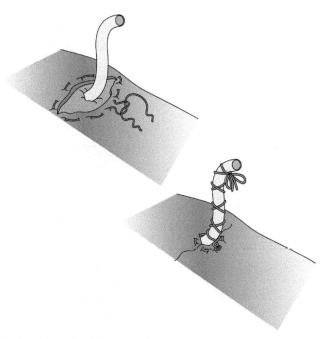

Figure 5.8 Securing a chest tube with a purse string suture.

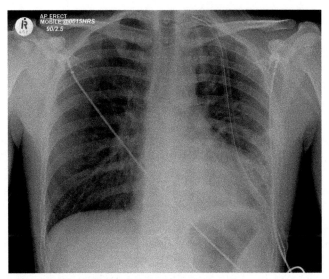

Figure 5.9 CXR showing a chest drain in position.

- The distal end of the drain tube must not be open to the environment, in order to prevent entrainment of air into the pleural space.
  - Attach to an underwater seal, a flap valve or sealed container.
- Low pressure suction can be applied to the drain to facilitate drainage.

Tips and advice

- Trocars are best used as stakes to support plants in your garden, not as chest drain insertion aids!

References/further reading

Laws D, Neville E, Duffy J (2003). British Thoracic Society guidelines for the insertion of a chest drain. *Thorax*, 58 (Supplement 2) p. ii53–ii59.

Seldinger chest drain insertion

Indications

- Pleural effusion.
- May be used for similar indications as a surgical drain but due to the smaller gauge of tubing may be less appropriate.

Contraindications

- As for surgical technique

Complications

- As for surgical technique

Equipment

- Portable ultrasound machine
- Basic dressing/minor procedure pack
- Antiseptic solution and sterile drapes
- Lidocaine 1–2%
- Seldinger kit chest drain 10–14 F
- Scalpel

- Skin suture
- Gauze
- Dressing
- Three–way tap
- Fluid drainage bag

Sites

- Posterior/Lateral approach.
  - Ideally the optimum insertion point should be located with the use of ultrasound.
    - Insert drain in intercostal space with greatest depth of pleural fluid underlying, and at furthest point from diaphragm to minimize potential trauma.
  - Ultrasound can either be used either by the operator at time of procedure or by a radiologist in advance with the appropriate insertion point marked.

Insertion technique

- Confirm diagnosis clinically and check position of diaphragm on CXR.
- Position patient.
  - This may require the patient to be placed in a more lateral position as the insertion site is often more posterior than the mid–axillary line (as in the surgical technique – see earlier).
  - Either place a pillow behind under the patient to help maintain position or ask an assistant to help roll the patient into a lateral position.
- Sterile technique.
- Identify the insertion point.
  - As guided by ultrasound.
- Infiltrate local anaesthetic.
- Avoiding lower margin of rib (where the neurovascular bundle runs), insert introducer needle at 90 degrees to skin, aspirating gently, until pleural fluid is aspirated.
- Remove syringe and insert guidewire through introducer needle.
- Remove introducer needle leaving guidewire in place.
- Insert dilator through skin over guidewire.
  - Passage of the dilator may be aided by a small skin incision with scalpel at insertion point of guidewire.
  - It is not necessary to insert dilator to the hilt (may cause trauma if inserted to hilt).
- Remove dilator ensuring the guidewire remains in place.
- Insert drain over guidewire.
- Remove guidewire.
- Attach three–way tap and fluid drainage bag to end of drain.
- Secure drain using skin suture as for surgical technique.
- Perform CXR to confirm placement (see Figure 5.10).

Important points/cautions

- If a radiologist assesses the insertion site in advance, then ensure that the patient is in the same position as when the ultrasound was performed in order to recreate the conditions at that time.
  - Ideally the person carrying out the procedure should be present during the ultrasound.

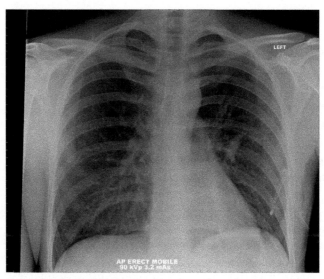

Figure 5.10 CXR of pigtail catheter in place.

- **Never** use a trocar to place a chest drain.
  - Blind insertion of a trocar can result in serious damage to lungs, blood vessels, heart and intra–abdominal organs.
  - Discard any trocar supplied with a drain before insertion.
- The distal end of the drain tube must not be open to the environment in order to prevent entrainment of air into the pleural space.
  - Attach to an underwater seal, a flap valve or sealed container.
- It is generally advised to remove a maximum of 1 litre of fluid at any one time and to do so slowly. Pulmonary oedema can result if large volumes are removed quickly.

References/further reading

Laws D, Neville E, Duffy J. BTS guidelines for the insertion of a chest drain. *Thorax* 2003; 58 (Supplement 2) p. ii53–ii59.

Removal of a chest drain

Indications

- Drain no longer draining air, blood or fluid.
- Full expansion of lung on CXR.
- No detectable air leak on coughing or valsalva manoeuvre.
- A more cautious approach is to clamp the drain for 24 hours to confirm there is no reaccumulation of air on a further CXR.

Contraindications

- Caution if patient on positive pressure ventilation (IPPV) as this tends to potentiate leaks.

Complications

- Reaccumulation of air, blood or fluid.
- Tension pneumothorax.

Equipment

- Equipment for sterile technique
- Sterile dressing pack/minor procedure pack
- Local anaesthetic with appropriate needle and syringe
- Suture material if purse string suture not already in situ
- Dressing

Removal technique

- Check X-ray.
- Clamp tube for 12–24 hours if appropriate.
- Clean and drape as for a sterile procedure
- Remove suture from around the tube.
- If purse string suture is in place cut and prepare suture for tying on tube removal.
- If no purse string suture is in present, place new purse string (see Figure 5.8) using local anaesthetic infiltration if appropriate.
- Remove tube at end of expiration and pull purse string suture tight.
- Place gauze swab firmly over the wound and secure the suture tightly.
- Cover with airtight dressing.
- Request a CXR.

Tips and advice

- Consider asking an assistant to remove the tube to facilitate closing the wound by securing the suture.

Pericardiocentesis

- Pericardiocentesis is a procedure that is rarely performed by anaesthetists.
- If required it will be in an acute setting where cardiac tamponade causes an acute fall in cardiac output or leads to cardiac arrest.

Indications
- Acute
  - Tamponade, postoperative or post–trauma
- Chronic
  - Pericardial effusions associated with infective, malignant or autoimmune conditions
    - Diagnosis and symptomatic relief
  - May present acutely and require acute drainage

Contraindications
- Absolute
  - None if being performed in the emergency setting
- Relative
  - Previous cardiac surgery
  - Inexperience with the technique

Complications
- Damage to the following structures during needle insertion (depending on approach).
  - Internal mammary artery.
  - Right/left ventricle puncture:
    - puncture of the thin walled right ventricle and atria can be catastrophic
    - puncture of the thick walled left ventricle may be better tolerated.
  - Atrial puncture.
  - Pleural puncture resulting in pneumothorax.
  - Coronary arteries.
- Arrhythmias.
  - Particularly bradycardias associated with pericardial puncture.
- Infection.

Equipment
- Resuscitation equipment
- Basic dressing pack/minor procedure pack
- Antiseptic solution
- Local anaesthetic
- Syringes and needles
- Pericardiocentesis pack
  - 10–15 cm needle, short bevelled
  - Guidewire
  - Catheter with side holes, usually 6–9 FG
- Scalpel
- Skin suture

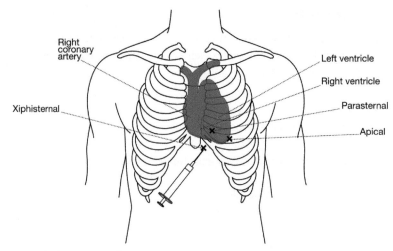

Figure 5.11 Surface anatomy of the heart with pericardiocentesis insertion points.

- Gauze
- Dressing

Sites

- There are a number of approaches described (see Figure 5.11).
  - Sub–xiphisternal:
    - palpate notch between xiphisternum and left costal margin
    - point needle at an angle of 45 degrees to the skin aiming towards the back of the left shoulder.
  - Anterior, parasternal (not described here).
  - Apical (not described here).

Insertion technique

- Ensure ECG monitoring and intravenous access are in place.
- Position patient in semi sitting position unless performed during resuscitation in which case do not move from the supine position.
- Aseptic technique.
- Infiltrate with local anaesthetic if appropriate.
- Identify landmarks as described above.
- Advance needle while gently aspirating on a connected syringe.
- Once fluid aspirated, either aspirate fluid through needle or insert catheter using Seldinger technique.
  - The introducing needle is narrow and can migrate easily from the pericardial space and catheter placement is recommended.
- If the catheter kit is supplied with a dilator, use it before threading the drain over the wire.
- Attach three–way tap to catheter and a 20 ml syringe, for aspiration, to the three–way tap.
- In case of acute tamponade, once catheter is in place aspirate as much blood as possible and assess patients condition.
- Secure catheter with tape or skin suture.

- Re–aspirate if fluid reaccumulates before performing or arranging appropriate definitive procedure.
- Request and review CXR to exclude complications of insertion e.g. pneumothorax.

Important points/cautions

- Ventricular arrhythmias on insertion suggest the needle is touching the ventricle. Withdrawal of the needle may resolve the arrhythmia.

Temporary cardiac pacing

- Temporary cardiac pacing can be achieved through a variety of means.
  - External pacing includes use of the fist, or percussion, for pacing in the immediate and emergency setting whilst organising transcutaneous pacing using a defibrillator and external, adhesive defibrillation pads.
  - Temporary internal (invasive) pacing involves the passage of a transvenous pacing wire via a central vein into the ventricle.

External temporary cardiac pacing: percussion pacing

Indications

- Profound bradycardia or complete atrioventricular block causing clinical cardiac arrest.

Contraindications

- Nil

Complications

- Failure to produce cardiac output.
  - This may be with or without the presence of QRS complexes.
- If no cardiac output consider alternative techniques or start CPR.

Equipment

- ECG monitoring
- Defibrillator
- Resuscitation drugs
- Resuscitation team aware

Sites

- Deliver blows over the precordium lateral to the lower left sternal edge.

Technique

- Ensure ECG monitoring, defibrillator and cardiac arrest team available.
- Identify landmark for blows (as above).
- Raise fist about 10 cm above the chest for each blow.
- Perform blow on precordium.
  - The force required initially is said to be that which would be tolerated by a conscious patient.
- If no QRS complex seen, try moving the site of contact around the precordium.
- If QRS complex seen reduce the force of the blows until the threshold is found.

Important points/cautions

- This technique is most likely to be successful when ventricular standstill is accompanied by continuing P wave activity.

- If QRS complexes and cardiac output not rapidly achieved then alternative resuscitation techniques should be performed.

Tips and advice

- If there is any doubt as to the diagnosis or success of pacing, advanced life support protocols should be commenced and CPR begun following the Resuscitation Council algorithms.

References/further reading

Resuscitation Council UK (2006) *Advanced Life Support. 5th edition.* Resuscitation Council (UK), London.

External temporary cardiac pacing: transcutaneous pacing

Indications

- Profound bradycardia or complete atrioventricular block causing clinical cardiac arrest.

Contraindications

- Nil

Complications

- Failure to produce cardiac output.
  - This may be with or without QRS complexes.
- If no cardiac output consider alternative techniques or start CPR.

Equipment

- Adhesive electrode pads for ECG monitoring, pacing, cardioversion and defibrillation
- Defibrillator
- Resuscitation drugs
- Resuscitation team aware

Sites

- The adhesive electrode pads can be placed in either of two positions.
  - Anteriorly in right pectoral and apical positions (see Figure 1.9).
    - Right pectoral pad placed to the right of the sternum below the clavicle.
    - Apical pad placed in the mid–axillary line, approximately level with the V6 electrode. Ensure clear of breast tissue.
  - Anterior–posterior position.
    - Anterior pad on the left anterior chest wall beside the sternum.
    - Posterior pad at the corresponding level to the anterior pad, between the lower part of the left scapula and the spine.

Technique

- Identify the application sites for the pads.
- If time remove chest hair to improve contact between skin and pad.
- Attach additional ECG monitoring if required in addition to the electrodes (depending on the equipment available).
- Select demand mode if available and adjust ECG gain to aid sensing of any intrinsic ECG activity.
- Select pacing rate.
- Increase pacing current slowly from the lowest level until pacing spikes on the ECG are followed by a QRS complex (typically between 50–100 mA).
  - Normally the muscles of the chest wall will contract with each impulse.
- If the maximum current is reached consider changing the pad positioning.
- If QRS complexes are seen on the ECG assess the patient's pulse. The presence of a pulse suggests successful pacing and the adequacy of cardiac output should be determined.
- If adequate cardiac output seek cardiology help immediately for consideration of insertion of a temporary pacing wire.

- **Remember**: if no QRS complexes are seen or if QRS complexes are present in the absence of a pulse, the patient should be treated as having a non−shockable rhythm cardiac arrest, and advanced life support and CPR should be commenced.

Important points/cautions

- The adhesive pads can be placed prior to high risk procedures as a precautionary manner in the event of a cardiac arrest, both for the possibility of pacing or for defibrillation depending on clinical indications.

Tips and advice

- If there is any doubt as to the diagnosis, availability of external pacing equipment or success of pacing, advanced life support protocols should be followed and CPR commenced following the Resuscitation Council algorithms.

Internal temporary cardiac pacing

- Insertion of a transvenous pacing wire will usually be performed by a cardiologist using a flotation catheter with or without X−ray guidance.
- It is likely to be performed once a patient has been stabilized after initial resuscitation and therefore the insertion of a temporary pacing wire is not going to be discussed here.
- Pacing wires are often encountered on ICU as well as in the theatre setting. We will discuss the daily management of a pacing wire (as should be conducted on ICU) and the common causes of failure of such a device.

Indications

- Bradycardias associated with a low cardiac output state.
- Tachyarrhythmias.
- Prophylactic pacing prior to anaesthesia in patients with a predisposition to bradyarrhythmias:
  - second degree heart block
  - third degree heart block
  - protocols vary locally regarding which patients should be paced prophylactically.

Contraindications

- No absolute contraindications depending on the clinical urgency.
  - Discuss locally.

Complications

- Threshold.
  - When inserted the aim is to achieve a threshold of less than 1 V, indicating good contact with the myocardium.
    - It is usual to pace the heart with 3−4 V stimulus.
  - Check the threshold at least daily to make sure that the output of the pacemaker is well above the threshold.
    - Loss of capture may occur if not.
  - To check.
    - Turn down the voltage to determine the point of loss of capture i.e. the point where a pacing spike no longer results in a QRS complex. Note the voltage and

then turn the voltage back to the original setting whilst confirming capture i.e. QRS complexes after pacing spike.

- An increasing threshold should prompt urgent referral to the cardiologists.
  - Loss of capture.
    - May be due to a high threshold. Immediately turn the output of the pacemaker to above the threshold until capture reestablished.
      - Refer to cardiologists.
- Electrode displacement.
  - Loss of contact with myocardium.
  - Perforation of right ventricle.
- Loss of electrical continuity.
  - Loss of electrical supply to pacing unit.
  - Loose connections between leads and pacemaker.

Chapter 6
Abdominal Procedures

Nasogastric and nasojejunal tube placement

- A wide variety of tubes are available for passing via the nose (or mouth) down the oesophagus and into the stomach.
- Single lumen, double lumen, fine–bore feeding tubes, and large–bore orogastric tubes are all available.
- Can be used to drain stomach contents, or to administer drugs, feed, or contrast agents.
- Gastric lavage is rarely performed nowadays, but would necessitate that passage of a nasogastric (NG) or orogastric tube.

Nasogastric tubes

Indications

- Aspiration of gastric contents for diagnostic (e.g. in suspected gastrointestinal (GI) haemorrhage) or therapeutic purposes.
  - Bowel obstruction.
  - Ileus.
  - Sepsis.
- Intra– or postoperatively where ileus may be expected to occur, or to facilitate surgery in laparoscopic procedures where a decompressed stomach is needed.
- Preoperative decompression of the stomach to reduce the risk of aspiration.
- Administration of drugs in patients unable to swallow.
- Administration of enteral feed.
- Gastric lavage (rarely used nowadays).
- Administration of radio–opaque contrast agent in X–ray studies of the upper gastrointestinal tract.
- Warm or cold fluid can be passed via a NG tube to aid aggressive warming (e.g. in hypothermia) or aggressive cooling (e.g. in malignant hyperpyrexia).

Contraindications

- NG tubes should **never** be inserted in patients with confirmed or suspected base of skull fracture.
  - There is a risk of passing the tube into the cranial vault.
  - An orogastric tube should be inserted instead.
  - NG tubes are associated with infection in the nasopharynx and could predispose to meningitis if open skull base fracture is present.
- Coagulopathy.
  - Trauma often accompanies NG tube insertion and bleeding from the nasal mucosa can be torrential.
  - Trauma to the oesophageal and gastric mucosa can also occur leading to GI haemorrhage.
- Care should be taken when inserting NG tubes in patients with a reduced conscious level, as vomiting can occur which increases the risk of aspiration. NG tubes in situ can disrupt the integrity of the lower oesophageal sphincter leading to reflux
  - Consideration should be given to protecting the patient's airway prior to NG tube insertion (i.e. intubation).
- Passage of NG tubes in patients with known or suspected oesophageal varices can lead to bleeding.

- Consultation with a senior physician should occur before passing a NG tube in patients with oesophageal strictures, or with previous oesophagectomy.

Complications

- Trauma
  - Nasal
  - Pharyngeal
  - Oesophageal
  - Gastric
  - Creation of false mucosal passage
- Bleeding
- Infection
  - Obstruction of nasal sinus drainage and nasal mucosal damage can lead to secondary sepsis.
- Vomiting
- Aspiration of gastric contents
- Misplacement of the tube
  - Tracheal or bronchial placement can be disastrous if feed or drugs are administered.
  - Cranial placement through basal skull fracture.
  - Placement in the oesophagus rather than the stomach, can lead to regurgitation and aspiration of administered substances.
- Blockage of the tube
  - This also increases the risk of aspiration.

Equipment

- A nasogastric tube of appropriate size for the desired purpose.
  - 14 FG is adequate for general gastric decompression.
  - Fine−bore tubes (usually 8 FG) are preferred for long−term feeding.
    - Fine−bore tubes usually have a guidewire in the lumen, which aids passage, but this needs to be removed prior to commencement of feeding.
  - Refrigerated NG tubes are stiffer and may be easier to pass.
    - In conscious patients, a floppy tube is just as easy to pass and is not as uncomfortable.
- Lubricating jelly (water soluble) or 2% lidocaine gel.
- Water +/− drinking straw for insertion in conscious patients.
- 50 ml **bladder** syringe.
- Stethoscope.
- Litmus paper.
- Adhesive tape.
- In anaesthetized patients:
  - laryngoscope (checked)
  - Magill's forceps.

Sites

- Right or left nostril.
  - Choice of side should be influenced by presence of deformities or blockages.

- Tubes may be passed orally.
  - Less well tolerated in conscious patients.
  - Preferred route in head injury and neurosurgical patients.

Insertion technique

- Awake patients should be in the sitting position if possible.
  - Gain informed consent from awake patients.
- Unconscious patients will be in the supine position.
- Examine the nostrils (ask patient to sniff through each in turn) and choose the most patent nostril.
- Wear gloves.
  - Aseptic technique is not needed.
  - Gloves will protect **you**.
- Lubricate the tube liberally with jelly.
  - Use lidocaine gel (2%) for conscious patients.
- The distance from the nose to the stomach can be estimated by placing the tube tip at the patient's earlobe and extending the tube via the bridge of the nose to the xiphoid process.
  - Make a note of this distance, or mark it with tape.
- Pass the tube horizontally into the nostril.
  - Note the direction is horizontal and **not** up into the nose.
- Pass the tube gently back into the nose.
- In conscious patients:
  - ask the patient to swallow repeatedly
  - consider asking the patient to suck some water from a straw, hold it in their mouth and swallow it when asked
  - swallowing increases the chances of the tube passing into the oesophagus.
- In anaesthetized/unconscious patients (see Figure 6.1):
  - an endotracheal tube should already be in situ, however some anaesthetists prefer placing an NG tube **before** tracheal intubation in elective surgical cases
  - perform laryngoscopy whilst inserting the NG tube into the nose in a direction parallel with the floor of the nose/palate
  - when the NG tube becomes visible in the mouth, stop advancing and take hold of the tip with some Magill's forceps
  - using the Magill's forceps pass the tube bit–by–bit into the oesophagus
  - alternatively use a cold tube: look at the curvature of the tube and insert it so the curvature would point cephalad hence keeping it posterior as it is inserted, then grip the valeculae with the other hand to close them and advance the tube gently down into the oesophagus (watch for any signs of coiling).
- When the tube has been inserted to the predetermined depth, attach 50 ml bladder syringe and attempt to aspirate gastric contents.
  - Any contents aspirated should be tested with litmus paper and should be acidic in pH.
- It is not always possible to aspirate any fluid, in which case 5–10 ml of air can be injected down the tube whilst auscultating over the stomach.
  - Obvious gurgling is heard over the stomach with correct placement.
- Secure the tube with tape on the nose.

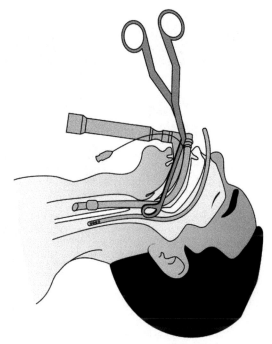

Figure 6.1 NG tube insertion technique with laryngoscope and Magill's forceps.

- With fine–bore tubes, **leave the guidewire in situ** until correct positioning has been confirmed according to departmental protocol.
- Correct position should be confirmed with a CXR (see Figures 6.2 and 6.3) if:
  ○ a fine–bore tube has been used

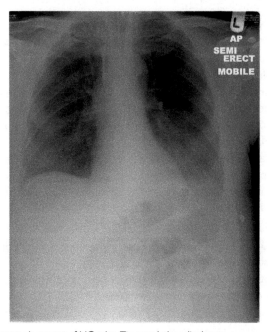

Figure 6.2 CXR of correct placement of NG tube. Tip seen below diaphragm.

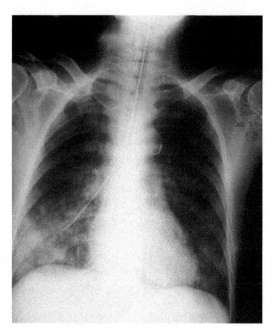

Figure 6.3 CXR of incorrect placement of NG tube in patients lungs. Ensure the tip of the NG tube is seen below the diaphragm.

- the patient has a chest or abdominal injury
- the patient is unconscious (**not** in elective surgical cases)
- there is **any** doubt about the position of the tube.
- With fine–bore tubes remove the wire when correct position is confirmed.

Important points/cautions
- Passage of NG tubes can be incredibly difficult.
- Assistance from experienced nurses may be invaluable in awake patients.
- Avoid repeated attempts as trauma is likely to occur.
  - **Ask for help** if you are finding it difficult to pass the tube.
- Passage of the tube into the airway will cause coughing and respiratory compromise in awake patients. Passage into the oesophagus will cause gagging.
  - Do not continue advancing the tube if the patient is coughing or becomes distressed.
- NG tubes can be passed into the airway even in intubated patients.
  - This will be evident as a leak around the cuff of an TT.
  - If this occurs, withdraw the NG tube **carefully** whilst holding the TT in place so as not to inadvertently extubate the patient.

Tips and advice
- Advancing the NG tube during expiration (in awake and unconscious patients) may help to avoid tracheal placement.
- In awake patients the oropharynx and nostril can be sprayed with 10% lidocaine.
- Do not use excessive force during insertion.
  - If resistance is encountered then consider removal and reinsertion.
    - False passages can be created.

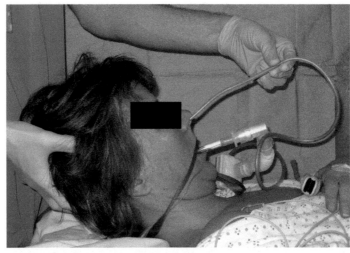

Figure 6.4 NG tube insertion technique. Flexing neck and head, and using the natural curvature of the NG tube. Greatest successful placement when NG tube cold and therefore more rigid.

- Fine−bore tubes have a guidewire in situ and this can cause severe trauma or perforation if excessive force is used.
- In awake patients:
  ○ if the patient (or you) becomes distressed, then abandon the procedure and reattempt later on or ask for help from a senior colleague.
- In intubated patients:
  ○ head flexion may aid passage (see Figure 6.4).
  ○ grasping the thyroid cartilage and pulling it anteriorly may aid passage (see Figure 6.5).

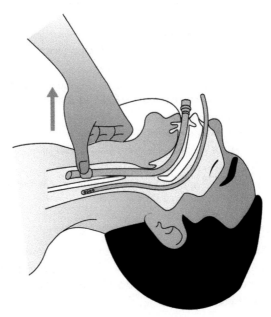

Figure 6.5 NG tube insertion technique. Thyroid traction.

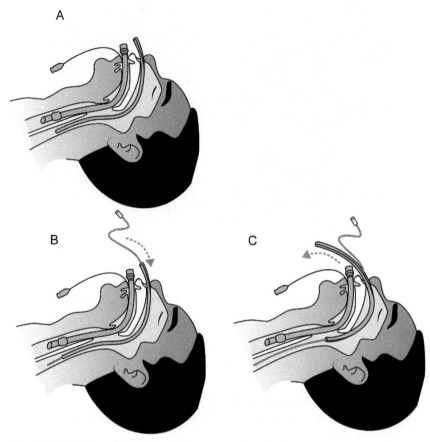

Figure 6.6 NG tube insertion technique. Split naso–oesophageal tube.

- ○ NG tubes may be inserted without the use of a laryngoscope but this becomes a blind procedure and trauma is more likely, as is misplacement
- ○ use of a split nasal tube may be of use (see Figure 6.6).
  - Pass a size 6 – 6.5 tube, which has been split longitudinally along its entire length, into the nostril (**after endotracheal intubation**).
  - Pass the tube into the oesophagus.
  - The NG tube is then passed through the split tube.
  - Once the NG tube is confirmed in the stomach, the split tube can be removed leaving the NG tube in situ.
- ○ Very occasionally the cuff of the TT may be obstructing passage of the NG tube, and temporary deflation will aid insertion.

Nasojejunal tubes

- Nasojejunal (NJ) tubes allow feeding directly into the small bowel.
- NJ tubes are useful if impaired gastric emptying (indicated by large aspirates with NG feeding) is occurring, with resistance to prokinetic agents.
- Also useful in pancreatitis.

- Spontaneous passage of NJ tubes through the pylorus is rare, and may be increased by the administration of prokinetics such as erythromycin, and by manipulation of patient position.
  - Insertion technique is the same as for NG tubes but the calculated insertion depth is greater.
- NJ tubes can only be reliably inserted to the correct position with endoscopic or fluoroscopic guidance.
- Correct placement should be confirmed with X−ray prior to starting feeding.
- NJ tubes **do not** reduce the risk of aspiration.

Sengstaken–Blakemore and Minnesota tube placement

- These are tubes which are used to apply pressure to oesophageal varices, thereby tamponading the vessels and reducing haemorrhage.
- The Sengstaken–Blakemore tube is a large triple lumen tube with two balloons – one gastric and one oesophageal. Two lumens exist to supply the balloons, while the third enables drainage of the stomach.
- The Minnesota tube differs in that it has a further lumen which can be used to drain the oesophagus – The Minnesota tube is now most commonly used but, confusingly, is often incorrectly referred to as a Sengstaken–Blakemore tube.
- Oesophageal varices occur where the portal and systemic circulations anastomose, at the lower end of the oesophagus.
- The oesophagus extends from the cricoid cartilage at C6, to the gastro–oesophageal junction at T10.
  - This is a distance of around 25 cm in most adults.
- See Figure 6.7.

Indications

- Bleeding from oesophageal varices of the lower oesophagus and gastro–oesophageal junction.
  - Insertion of these tubes is a **temporary** measure which is used to control bleeding, 'buying time' in which the patient can be resuscitated if necessary and more definitive treatment can be instituted.

Contraindications

- The presence of a significant hiatus hernia is a **relative** contraindication.

Complications

- Pulmonary aspiration – relatively high risk during insertion.
  - Consider pre–procedure intubation if:
    - distressed, anxious or uncooperative patient
    - significant instability (cardiovascular, respiratory)

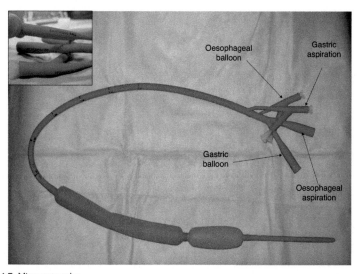

Oesophageal balloon

Gastric aspiration

Gastric balloon

Oesophageal aspiration

Figure 6.7 Minnesota tube.

- sedation should **never** be given to facilitate tube insertion **but** anaesthesia might be safer for safe insertion and use.
- If the gastric balloon is inflated in the oesophagus, this may result in oesophageal rupture.
- Prolonged/heavy traction can cause nasal ulceration within hours.
  - This may also lead to migration of the tube into the hypopharynx, with the potential to cause airway obstruction.
- Prolonged use with pressure on the oesophageal mucosa may lead to mucosal necrosis and ulceration.
  - This complication can be avoided by deflating the oesophageal balloon for a few minutes every 6 hours.

Equipment

- Sengstaken–Blakemore or Minnesota tube
- High flow suction available and working
- 50 ml bladder syringe
- 10% lidocaine spray
- Lubricating jelly (water–soluble)
- Sphygmomanometer and three–way tap
- Sterile saline (if using saline to inflate the balloons)
- Four clamps (for clamping the tube)
- Traction weights (300 g)
  - A bag of saline containing 300 ml of fluid can be used

Sites

- Sengstaken–Blakemore and Minnesota tubes are usually inserted via the nose.
- Oral insertion is also possible.
- The nasal route is more uncomfortable **during** insertion, but less uncomfortable when the tube is in situ.

Insertion technique

- If the patient is vomiting and a decision has been made **not** to intubate, then insertion in the lateral decubitus position is safest.
- Check the tube prior to insertion.
  - Each balloon should be inflated and checked for leaks.
  - The lumina should be checked for patency.
  - The volume required to fill each balloon should be noted.
    - It is most important to know the volume of the oesophageal balloon.
    - The sphygmomanometer can be attached to the pressure port of each balloon, and the pressure measured after each 50 ml increment of air or saline is instilled.
- A refrigerated tube may be easier to insert.
- Anaesthetize the naso– and oropharynx with 10% lidocaine spray.
- Lubricate the tube liberally with water soluble jelly.
- Identify the most patent nostril if using the nasal route (see section on NG tubes).
- Advance the tube nasally or orally.
  - In many patients the nasal route will not be tolerated and the oral route should be used.
- In conscious patients, ask them to swallow as the tube is advanced.

- If the patient vomits, place in the lateral position and have an assistant help with suctioning vomitus from the mouth.
- The tube should be advanced to a depth of around 50 cm.
- Position should be checked by injecting 5–10 ml of air into the gastric port whilst auscultating over the stomach.
- If correct position is verified, then inflate the gastric balloon.
  - Inflate using air or saline.
  - Approximately 250 ml for a Sengstaken–Blakemore tube, and around 400–500 ml for a Minnesota tube.
  - The pressures measured after each 50 ml increment should be **no more** than 15 mmHg greater than the pressures measured for the same values when checking the balloon.
    - Higher pressures indicate that the balloon is in the oesophagus or duodenum and needs repositioning.
- Once the gastric balloon is fully inflated, close the gastric inflation port and clamp it.
- Pull the tube back gently until the gastric balloon lodges against the gastro–oesophageal junction. This will be felt as an obvious resistance.
- The tube should then be taped to the nose.
- Request an abdominal X–ray to check the position of the gastric balloon.
- Next, inflate the oesophageal balloon.
  - The balloon should be inflated to a pressure of 25–35 mmHg (roughly 100 ml volume).
  - The pressure should be checked using the sphygmomanometer attached to the oesophageal pressure port.
  - Clamp the inflation port after inflation.
  - The pressure should be checked regularly at 4 hourly intervals.
- Traction should be applied to the tube.
  - The traction weight should be roughly 300 g.
  - A 300 ml bag of saline is useful as a weight.
  - Skin traction is an alternative.
    - The tube is taped securely to the patient's face.
- See Figure 6.8.

Important points/cautions

- The insertion of a tamponading tube to control bleeding from oesophageal varices is only a temporary measure. Definitive treatment should be instituted when possible and the case should be discussed with gastroenterology and general surgical teams.
- Intermittent suction should be applied to the gastric port.
  - Continuous suction should be applied to the oesophageal suction port (Minnesota tube only).
- Necrosis of the oesophageal wall is a significant risk.
  - The pressure in the oesophageal balloon should be maintained at the lowest level that is successful in controlling bleeding.
  - The oesophageal balloon should be intermittently deflated, e.g. for 5 minutes every 6 hours.
- After 24 hours, the oesophageal balloon should be deflated and traction removed.
  - If this does not lead to bleeding, leave the tube in situ for 24 hours prior to deflating the gastric balloon and removal.

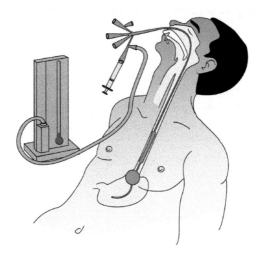

Figure 6.8 Minnesota gastric balloon in place.

○ If bleeding does occur after oesophageal balloon deflation, then the balloon should be reinflated and the tube left in situ for another 12–24 hours.

　▪ An urgent surgical opinion should be sought.

Tips and advice

● A stiffer tube may be easier to insert.

　○ Use a tube which has been in the refrigerator.

● If the patient is vomiting profusely, is agitated and uncooperative, or if there is any depression of conscious level then intubation to protect the airway **before** insertion of the tamponading tube is advisable.

● Contrast media can be mixed with saline to be used in balloon inflation.

　○ This allows easier visualization of balloon position on X–ray.

● During oesophageal balloon inflation, watch for any signs of respiratory compromise or complaints of pain.

● Cardiac arrhythmias can occur as the oesophageal balloon is inflated.

Urethral catheterization

- Commonly performed procedure.
- Involves the passage of a rubber, silicone or plastic catheter into the bladder, via the urethra.
  - The material used influences the length of time that a catheter can remain *in situ* (see Table 6.1).
- Urinary catheters have an inflatable balloon (of varying size) distally, to retain the catheter in the bladder.
- Urinary catheters have varying numbers of drainage/instillation channels.
- Male catheterization is usually performed by medical staff. Nurses usually catheterize female patients.
- This section will therefore focus on insertion of a urinary catheter in a male.

Indications

- Monitoring urine output:
  - in critically ill patients
  - during long surgical procedures
  - in haemodynamically unstable patients.
- Monitoring:
  - Intra-abdominal pressure
- Urinary retention:
  - secondary to prostatic hypertrophy
  - secondary to neurological disorders
  - during/following spinal or epidural anaesthesia.
- In some cases of urinary incontinence.

Contraindications

- Suspected traumatic rupture of the urethra
  - Indicated in patients with:
    - history of trauma to pelvis
    - high−riding prostate
    - blood at the urethral meatus
    - scrotal bruising.
- If the patient has a sensitivity to latex then use a 100% silicone catheter.

Complications

- Failure to pass the catheter is the commonest complication.
  - More likely in male patients due to the longer urethra and presence of the prostate gland.
  - Urethral strictures, prostatic hypertrophy and hypertrophy of the bladder neck increase the chance of failure.

Table 6.1 Maximum times before routine change necessary for various types of catheter (Manufacturer's recommendations should always be followed)

Material	Maximum duration of insertion
PVC (plastic)Specialist urology procedures	14 days
PTFE (Teflon coated latex)	28 days
Hydrogel coated (e.g. biocath)	12 weeks
All (pure 100%) silicone	12 weeks

- Trauma to the urethra, prostate and bladder.
  - This can occur on insertion **or** in traumatic removal of a catheter with the balloon inflated.
- Haemorrhage.
- Creation of a false passage.
- Urinary tract infection (UTI).
  - More common with long–term catheterization.
- Urethral stricture.
  - A late complication.
  - More likely in traumatic insertions.
- Blocked catheter.
  - May lead to 'bypassing' – where urine leaks out of the urethra from around the catheter.

Equipment

- Most hospitals have ready–prepared catheterization packs.
- If a pack is not available, then the following should be prepared.
  - Sterile drape/drapes
  - Cotton wool balls
  - Gauze swabs
  - Disposable plastic forceps
  - 1% lidocaine gel (10 ml)
  - Disposable dish to collect urine
  - Appropriate size syringe containing sterile water (NICE guidelines 2006) to inflate the balloon.
    - Most commonly used catheters have 10 ml balloons.
    - Some catheters (e.g. three–way irrigation catheters) have larger volume balloons.
    - Always check the correct balloon volume prior to starting.
  - Antiseptic cleaning solution.
  - Appropriate size catheter.
    - This will depend on local guidelines and the intended use
    - Catheters are sized using the Charriere gauge system (Ch or F), where 1 F/Ch = 0.33 mm.
    - Catheter sizes typically used for surgical patients would be 12 – 16 F.
    - Male catheters are longer than those intended for use in females (typically 40–44 cm compared to 26 cm). Ensure you choose the correct one!
  - Sterile gloves
  - Urine collection bag
    - Various types exist
    - If urine output volume is to be measured then a collection bag with an appropriate measuring chamber should be used, e.g. urometer, hourly–urine bags.

Sites

- Urethral catheterization only takes place via the urethra.
- Catheterization of the bladder can take place via the abdominal wall in patients where urethral passage is difficult or impossible. This is 'supra–pubic catheterization' and is not covered within this book, as it is performed by urologists.

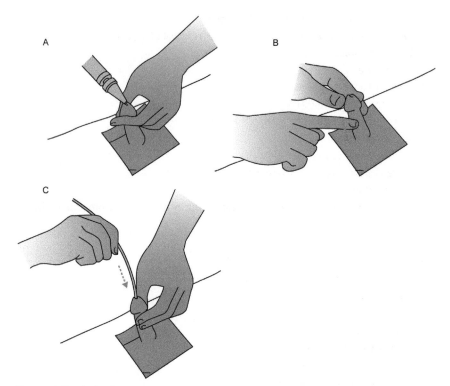

Figure 6.9 Urethral catheterization in a male.

Insertion technique

- This refers to **male** catheterization (see Figure 6.9).
- Inform the patient about the procedure and gain consent.
- Consider the need for antibiotic prophylaxis/cover.
- Protect bedding/mattress with pads.
- The patient should be in the supine position with his legs slightly apart.
- Prepare the equipment listed above on a sterile trolley.
  - Soak the cotton wool balls in antiseptic solution.
  - Partially open the packet containing the catheter, so that the catheter can be inserted with one hand later on.
  - Draw up the correct volume of sterile water for balloon inflation (if necessary).
- Wash hands.
- Create a sterile field and maintain aseptic technique throughout.
  - Use drapes to achieve this. Either a single fenestrated drape, or a combination of drapes to create the field around the penis.
- Wrap a sterile swab around the penis.
- Retract the foreskin (if present).
- While holding the sterile swab around the penis in one hand, cleanse the glans penis with the cotton wool balls soaked in antiseptic solution using the other hand.
- With the penis extended, gently insert the nozzle of the tube of lidocaine gel into the urethral meatus.
  - Squeeze the contents of the lidocaine gel tube into the urethra.
  - Remove the tube from the meatus.

- Gently squeeze the distal end of the penis to prevent the gel from leaving the urethra.
  - This should be continued for 2 minutes in awake patients, but this is not necessary in anaesthetized patients.
- With the penis extended, insert the end of the catheter into the meatus.
- Gently feed the catheter into the urethra, holding the catheter through the packaging.
- If the catheter packaging is sticking to the catheter, then the hand holding the penis can be used to grip the catheter inside the urethra as the packaging is shaken free from the catheter with the other hand.
- The catheter should pass easily and without too much resistance.
- Continue to feed the catheter into the urethra to the bifurcation point.
- Urine should flow.
  - Place the external end of the catheter in a dish to collect the urine.
  - This does not always happen at once as the bladder may be empty or the lidocaine gel can temporarily obstruct the flow.
- Inflate the balloon with the correct volume of sterile water.
- Attach the closed drainage system.
- Replace the retracted foreskin (if applicable).
- Document the procedure in the notes/chart.

Important points/cautions

- In conscious patients, use plenty of lidocaine gel and give it adequate time to work (2–5 minutes).
- Some catheters have their own closed systems for inflation of the balloon, meaning that additional sterile water is not needed.
- Do not persist with repeated attempts at catheterization if an obstruction cannot be passed.
- If unable to pass a catheter with gentle pressure, seek advice and assistance from a urologist.
- Catheter introducers can cause severe trauma in unskilled hands; they should **only** be used by specialists with appropriate training.
- Patients having a catheter inserted should be assessed for the need for antibiotic prophylaxis in accordance with local guidelines and policies.

Tips and advice

- A little resistance is usually encountered when the tip of the catheter encounters the external bladder sphincter.
  - Asking the patient to cough, take a deep breath or to strain as if voiding, may help to ease passage.
- Keeping the penis in an 'extended' position makes passage easier.
- If urine does not flow immediately following insertion, gentle pressure on the abdominal wall overlying the bladder may help.

Abdominal paracentesis

- Abdominal paracentesis involves the removal of fluid from the peritoneal cavity.
- It can be either a single 'tap' to obtain samples for analysis to aid in diagnosis, or the insertion of a drain as a therapeutic procedure.

Indications

- Diagnostic
  - In new-onset ascites:
    - to determine aetiology
    - to differentiate an exudate from a transudate
    - to detect cancerous cells.
  - To diagnose or exclude spontaneous bacterial peritonitis (SBP).
- As a therapeutic procedure to relieve the problems associated with ascites:
  - prevent respiratory compromise secondary to abdominal distension
  - improve patient comfort
  - reduce intra-abdominal pressure.

Contraindications

- Patient refusal.
- All are relative, but will make the procedure more hazardous:
  - coagulopathy
  - pregnancy
  - abdominal scarring
  - infection over the abdominal wall
  - gaseous distension of the bowel
  - uncooperative, confused patient.

Complications

- Abdominal paracentesis is a relatively safe procedure.
- However, it is usually performed on sick patients.
- In the UK, the risk of a serious complication is approx. 1 in 1000 (see 2006 Guidelines on the Management of Ascites in Cirrhosis, British Society of Gastroenterology)
- Complications include:
  - significant bleeding
  - infection
  - renal failure
  - hyponatraemia
  - hepatic encephalopathy
  - bowel or bladder perforation
  - persistent leakage of ascites from aspiration site.

Equipment

- Sterile gloves and gown
- Needles
  - 25G for local anaesthetic infiltration
  - 22 or 21G for aspiration (if performing a diagnostic tap)
  - 1% or 2% lidocaine (5 ml)

- Syringes
  - 5 ml for local anaesthetic
  - 20 ml for aspiration of samples
- Skin preparation such as 2% chlorhexidene in alcohol
  - Follow local guidelines
- Sterile drapes
- If continued drainage of large volumes is intended then an indwelling drain should be chosen
  - A 'pigtail' drainage catheter is the best choice
- A closed drainage bag with an appropriate connector to attach to the drain
- Sterile specimen pots (2–3) and blood culture bottles
- Suture (2.0 silk) and/or adhesive tape
- Gauze swabs (sterile)

Sites

- The ideal site is controversial (see Figure 6.10).
- The site should be over an area of dullness to percussion.
  - Patient position can be modified to 'move' the ascitic fluid thereby making drainage easier.
- The chosen site should be influenced by a thorough examination of the patient's abdomen.
  - Avoid obvious vessels, solid tumour masses, sites of infection and scars.
- Bowel tends to 'float' on ascitic fluid, therefore aspiration performed anteriorly will be more likely to damage bowel.
- Either chose:
  - a point level with the umbilicus, 2–3 cm lateral to a line passing through the mid–inguinal point (see Figure 6.10)
  - a midline site 2 cm below the umbilicus through the linea alba.
- Ultrasound is being used more and more to help choose the optimum site for aspiration, and to guide drain insertion.

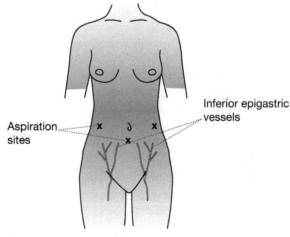

Figure 6.10 Sites for peritoneal aspiration (x).

Insertion technique

- Ascitic tap
  - Explain the procedure to the patient, including the risks, and obtain consent.
  - Place the patient in the supine position.
    - The head of the bed can be elevated to move the fluid to the lower abdomen.
    - Patients with smaller volumes of ascites can be tilted laterally (left or right) to enable bowel to float away from the fluid level.
  - Ensure the patient has emptied their bladder (if not catheterized).
  - Clean the skin with an antiseptic solution.
  - Infiltrate the skin and deeper layers with local anaesthetic.
    - Use the 25G needle for the skin.
    - Then change to a 21 or 22G needle for the deeper layers.
  - Move the needle deeper and 'draw–back' as you go until fluid is aspirated.
  - Ascitic fluid is typically straw–coloured.
  - Attach a new, sterile 20 ml syringe and aspirate 20 ml of fluid (or as much as can be aspirated).
  - Withdraw the syringe and needle.
  - Apply an absorbent dressing over the puncture site.
  - Divide the sampled fluid between the sterile pots and the two blood culture bottles.
    - Samples should be sent for:
      - protein and LDH content – biochemistry
      - microscopy, culture and sensitivities – microbiology
      - stain and culture for AFBs – microbiology
      - cytology – if a malignant process is suspected.
- Drainage of ascites
  - The insertion sites are the same as for a tap.
  - The insertion technique is the same as above.
  - When fluid is aspirated with the 21 or 22G needle whilst infiltrating local anaesthetic, remove the needle and syringe.
  - Then take the drain with the metal introducer needle in situ.
  - Attach a 5 ml syringe to the port of the drain needle.
  - Insert the drain/needle through the skin at the same site as before.
  - Pass through the deeper layers, constantly aspirating on the syringe until fluid is again aspirated freely.
  - As if inserting a venous cannula (cannula over needle), slide the drain catheter over the introducer needle, ensuring the needle is held in place.
    - The drain catheter should pass freely.
    - If resistance is encountered, withdraw, reinsert the introducer needle and move deeper until fluid if freely aspirated again.
  - Insert the drain catheter as far as it will go.
  - Take samples (as above) using a 20 ml syringe attached to the drain.
  - Attach the drainage system and bag to the drain.
    - Ensure fluid is draining freely.
  - Fix the drain to the abdominal wall **securely**, using either tape, sutures or both.
  - Dress the site with gauze and a transparent dressing.

Important points/cautions

- Prior to performing paracentesis, certain investigations should be carried out and the results checked.
  - FBC and clotting screen.
    - Consider correction of clotting/thrombocytopenia.
  - Abdominal USS.

Beware hypotension.

- Drainage of ascites.
  - Expert opinion is that swift drainage 'to dryness' is safest.
  - All ascitic fluid should be drained as rapidly as possible over 1–4 hours.
  - If the patient develops symptoms related to hypotension:
    - the BP should be monitored closely
    - the drainage rate can be slowed or stopped (clamp)
    - when drainage ceases the drain should be removed and the wound sutured if necessary, and dressed.
  - Large volume drainage (5 litres or more) can lead to post–paracentesis circulatory dysfunction (PPCD), characterized by:
    - hyponatraemia
    - azotaemia (renal failure and uraemia)
    - increased plasma rennin.
  - Current guidelines (Moore 2006) suggest that drainage of 5 litres or more should be accompanied by plasma expansion using 20% albumin.
    - The ratio is 8 g albumin per litre of ascites drained.
- Drains left *in situ* for longer than 6–8 hours may lead to increased risk of infection.
- In most situations, ascites will tend to reform and repeat drainage may be needed.

Tips and advice

- Incorporating a three–way tap into the drainage circuit makes it possible to take samples and flush drains.
  - This makes the introduction of infection more of a problem and strict aseptic technique should be used.
- A 'Z' track technique used when inserting the drain can minimize fluid leakage after it is removed: the needle/drain is inserted initially perpendicular to the skin, then angled obliquely as it passes through deeper structures, then place perpendicular again as it passes through the peritoneum.
  - This means the peritoneal and skin wounds are not in line
- If drainage slows or ceases, the patient's position should be altered, moving them from left– to right–lateral to encourage more drainage.

References/further reading

Moore KP and Aithal GP. Guidelines on the Management of Ascites in Cirrhosis, British Society of Gastroenterology. *Gut.* 2006 Oct; 55 p. Suppl 6:vi1–vi12.

Chapter 7
Neurological and Related Procedures

Local anaesthesia

- Local anaesthetic should be used prior to painful invasive procedures.
- Anaesthesia of the skin can be achieved using topical preparations, (particularly useful in children) or by infiltrating tissues with local anaesthetic solutions using a small gauge needle.

Indications

- Prior to invasive procedures

Contraindications

- Allergy to local anaesthetic

Complications

- Local bleeding
- Accidental puncture of superficial structures i.e. veins, arteries, with haematoma formation
- Pain

Equipment

- Topical anaesthetic preparation
  - Topical cream
    - Ametop: Tetracaine 4% (amethocaine). Effective within 30 minutes for venepuncture and 45 minutes for venous cannulation. Remains effective for 4–6 hours
    - EMLA™: Lidocaine 2.5% and prilocaine 2.5%. Apply 1–5 hours before procedure. Not recommended in children under 1 month (risk of methaemoglobinaemia)
  - Occlusive dressing
- Local infiltration
  - Sterile swab for skin
  - Lidocaine – 1 or 2% with or without adrenaline (epinephrine) 1:100000 – 1:200000
  - 2 or 5 ml syringe
  - 25G needle

Sites

- Dependent on procedure

Insertion technique

- Topical anaesthesia
  - Identify site for planned procedure.
  - Apply topical cream to skin.
  - Cover with occlusive dressing.
  - Leave in place until planned procedure takes place, or for recommended length of time dependent on cream used.
- Local infiltration
  - Lidocaine – 1 or 2%.
  - 2 or 5 ml syringe.
  - Aseptic technique.

○ Infiltrate local anaesthetic subcutaneously at the point where the subsequent procedure is planned.

■ Aim to raise a small subdermal "bleb" and wait for 30–60 seconds.

○ Massaging the area reduces any effect of the local anaesthetic distorting the anatomy prior to needle/cannula insertion.

○ Insert needle through the anaesthetized area.

Important points/cautions

• Warn the patient that the initial injection of local anaesthetic will sting briefly.

• Avoid using local anaesthetic with adrenaline (epinephrine) in any area involving end arteries i.e. fingers/toes as this risks vasoconstriction and digit ischaemia.

Tips and advice

• Try to avoid injecting the local anaesthetic directly over a blood vessel as this increases the chances of bleeding/haematoma formation.

Lumbar puncture

- Lumbar puncture (LP) involves accessing the subarachnoid space to obtain samples of cerebrospinal fluid (CSF).
- Samples can be sent for analysis to aid diagnosis.
- Anaesthetic staff are often asked to perform 'difficult' lumbar punctures due to their greater experience in accessing the subarachnoid space.

Indications

Lumbar puncture is indicated in the investigation of the following.

- Meningitis
- Subarachnoid haemorrhage (SAH), **if** CT scan of brain is normal
- Transverse myelitis
- Cerebral/parenchymal inflammation or infection
  - e.g. suspected multiple sclerosis, chronic infections (HIV, neurosyphilis)
- Demyelinating neuropathy
  - e.g. Guillain–Barre syndrome
- CSF disorders
  - e.g. benign intracranial hypertension, normal pressure hydrocephalus
- Chronic meningeal inflammation/infiltration
  - e.g. cancers, sarcoidosis

Also indicated as a therapeutic technique for:

- Removal of CSF to reduce ICP
- Injection of therapeutic agents into the CSF

Contraindications

- **If in doubt, perform a CT scan of the brain first to exclude a space–occupying lesion or obstructed CSF system**.
- Patient refusal.
- Main contraindication is the presence of an intracranial mass.
  - LP may cause trans–tentorial herniation (coning) and death.
  - Not all intracranial masses cause papilloedema, and so the absence of this sign does not guarantee a safe LP.
- Raised ICP for any reason.
- Focal neurological signs or symptoms.
  - These may be due to an underlying mass lesion.
- Coagulopathy or thrombocytopenia.
  - Different institutions and physicians have different 'cut–offs' in terms of the lowest platelet count at which they would perform a LP. This is usually in the range of $50 – 100 \times 10^9/L$. **If the platelet count is less than $100 \times 10^9/l$, discuss with your consultant.**

Complications

- Post dural–puncture headache (PDPH)
  - See later section on spinal anaesthesia.
  - Occurs in up to 25% of LPs.
  - Incidence can be reduced by use of smaller gauge, atraumatic spinal needles, keeping patient supine post–procedure, and encouraging fluid intake.

- Trauma to nerve roots
  - Rare (1:2,000 – 1:15,000).
  - Increased incidence if needle doesn't remain in the midline.
  - Patient may complain of pain or paraesthesiae in the leg(s).
  - **Withdraw** needle if patient complains of neurological symptoms, and if persistent call for senior assistance.
- Bleeding
  - Minor bleeding is not uncommon, as in 'bloody tap.'
  - Coagulopathy increases the risk of subarachnoid or subdural haemorrhage and paralysis due to haematoma formation.
- Coning
  - Tonsillar herniation may occur if LP is performed in a patient with raised ICP.
  - Risk reduced with a normal CT scan pre–procedure.
  - A rapid fall in the patient's GCS, new focal neurological signs, pupillary changes, haemodynamic disturbance (usually bradycardia and hypertension) would usually accompany coning.
    - Immediately call for help.
    - Resuscitate as per A, B, C.
    - Institute measures to reduce the ICP.
- Infection
  - Rare if **full** aseptic technique is employed.
  - CNS infection following LP can be devastating for the patient and the doctor.
  - Systemic sepsis in the patient may increase the risk of introducing bacteria into the CSF, and in these situations discussion with the physician in charge of the patient's care is mandatory.

Equipment

- Antiseptic solution
- 1% lidocaine and 25G needle for skin infiltration
- Spinal needle
  - Practice varies as to the needle size and type used.
    - The smaller the gauge, the less likely a dural puncture headache but the more likely that the procedure will be technically difficult and the flow of CSF may not be adequate for samples or ICP measurement.
    - The use of an introducer needle may help the insertion of smaller gauge needles.
  - Typically, a 22G or smaller Whitacre or Quincke needle is used.
- Manometer tubing
- 3 sterile bottles for collecting CSF samples
- Dressing

Sites/anatomical considerations

- Within the spinal canal the spinal cord extends down to L1–2.
- Below this extend the fimbriae, which are relatively mobile and therefore unlikely to be damaged by the introduction of a spinal needle. Therefore the L3/4 lumbar level is most frequently chosen to insert the needle.
  - This level can be identified determining the level of Tuffier's line, the line joining the posterior superior iliac spines, that overlies the L3/4 interspace or L4 vertebrae (Figure 7.2).

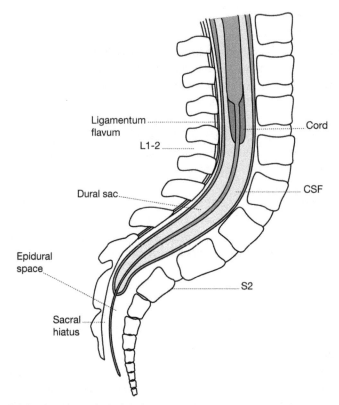

Figure 7.1 Lumbar spine and spinal cord anatomy.

Insertion technique

- Prepare equipment and explain procedure to patient.
- Position the patient (see next section and Figure 7.2).
- Identify posterior superior iliac spines, and the virtual line joining these points (Tuffier's line).
- Full aseptic technique.
- Infiltrate local anaesthetic.
- Stabilize skin over selected interspace using left hand (if right handed)
- Using a 22G needle or smaller insert needle at midpoint of L3/4 interspace and advance at slight cephalad angle.
- Needle will pass through skin, subcutaneous tissue, supraspinous ligament, interspinous ligaments, ligamentum flavum, and dura. A loss of resistance should be felt on passing through the ligamentum flavum and dura.
- Withdraw stylet and watch for CSF to flow down needle.
- Connect needle to the manometer and measure the pressure.
- Collect required specimens.
  - Microscopy and culture.
  - Examination for xanthochromia, protein and glucose.
  - Any special examinations i.e. immunological or viral studies or cytology.

- Withdraw needle.
- Apply dressing.

Important points/cautions

- Any pain, especially shooting pain into leg, suggests the needle is touching a nerve.
  - Needle should be withdrawn immediately.
- Blood in the needle hub on removal of the stylet often clears as CSF flows and does not require withdrawal of the needle. It will however affect the red blood cell count on microscopy!

Tips and advice

- If bone is encountered as the needle advances it is either too lateral or in the wrong vertical plane.
  - As a rule a slight cephalad approach, even in the lumbar area, is more likely to pass directly into the space.
  - If difficulty locating CSF then withdraw needle to skin and then redirect needle methodically, first aiming more cephalad then caudal.
  - If still unable withdraw needle completely and change skin insertion point by 1 cm and reattempt. If still difficulty try alternative interspace or call for senior help.
- The importance of good positioning should not be underestimated. An 'easy' back can become a very difficult lumbar puncture with poor positioning, as can a 'difficult' back be made into an easier lumbar puncture with good positioning.
- Use an introducer needle if using a spinal needle smaller than 24G.

Spinal anaesthesia

Indications

- Anaesthesia for operative intervention in the area which can be blocked by spinal anaesthesia.
  - Lower limb surgery
  - Lower abdominal surgery (inguinal hernia, caesarean section).
  - Perineal surgery.
- Analgesia for upper abdominal surgery or lower limb surgery in conjunction with general anaesthesia.

Contraindications

Absolute

- Raised ICP.
  - May result in the patient 'coning.'
    - See section on lumbar puncture.
- Systemic sepsis or local infection at puncture site.
  - Increased risk of subsequent epidural abscess formation or meningitis.
- Patient refusal.

Relative

- Known cardiovascular disease.
  - Especially aortic stenosis, mitral stenosis, pulmonary hypertension.
  - Conditions leading to a 'fixed' cardiac output.
- Previous back surgery.
  - Due to anticipated technical difficulty with procedure.
- Hypovolaemia.
  - Risk of exaggerated hypotension.
- Coagulopathy/thrombocytopenia.
  - Intra/extradural bleeding may occur, resulting in haematoma formation.
- Existing neurological deficit or disease.

Complications

- Failure to achieve an adequate block.
- Variable speed of onset resulting in haematoma formation:
  - hypotension
  - tachycardia
  - bradycardia associated with blockade of cardiac sympathetic fibres (above T5 level)
  - potential high block with phrenic nerve block or 'total spinal.'
- Loss of intercostal muscle strength with blocks higher than T10 resulting in sensation of dyspnoea.
- Post dural puncture headache.
- Backache.
- Urinary retention.
- Infection.
  - Meningitis or epidural abscess.
- Haematoma.
- Cranial nerve palsies.

Equipment

- Antiseptic solution
- 1% lidocaine and a 25G needle for skin infiltration
- 25G or 27G spinal needle with introducer
  - Most commonly, Whitacre atraumatic pencil–point needles are used
- Local anaesthetic +/− opiate to be injected
- Dressing

Sites and anatomical considerations

- Within the spinal canal the cord extends down to L1–2 level.
- Below this extend the fimbriae which are relatively mobile and therefore unlikely to be damaged by the introduction of a spinal needle. Therefore the L3/4 lumbar level is most frequently chosen to insert the needle.
- This level can be identified determining the level of Tuffier's line, the line joining the posterior superior iliac spines that overlies the L3/4 interspace or L4 vertebrae (see Figure 7.2).

Insertion technique

- Prepare equipment and explain procedure to patient.
- Attach patient to appropriate monitoring (see section on monitoring).
- Insert intravenous cannula and attach to intravenous fluid via giving set.
- Preload with fluid if appropriate.
- Position the patient (see Figures 7.3 and 7.4).
  - Ensure the operating table is flat and level with adequate lighting.
  - Position all equipment to be used within easy reach.
  - Anticipate the position required for the operator. This should be a comfortable, stable position, either kneeling, sitting or standing depending on preference (see Figure 7.4).

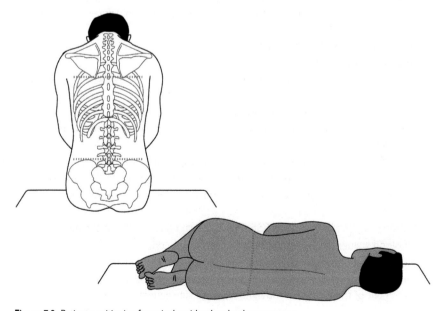

Figure 7.2 Patient positioning for spinal, epidural or lumbar puncture.

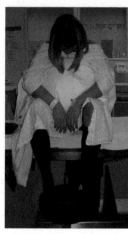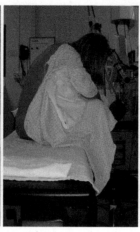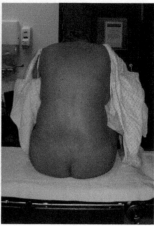

Figure 7.3 Positioning of patient for spinal anaesthesia (sitting).

○ Position patient sitting or lateral depending on preference.
  ■ Sitting: often easier the locate midline and therefore CSF, particularly in the obese.
    • Feet on stool, chin on chest, 'relax' shoulders and curved back (often aided by giving patient a pillow to hug).
  ■ Lateral: sometimes difficult to achieve level spine, parallel to bed complicating identification of the midline, especially in the obese.
    • Draw knees up towards chest (an assistant helps with positioning), chin on chest, curving back (see Figure 7.7).
• Identify the posterior superior iliac spines and the virtual line joining these points (Tuffier's line).
  ○ Research has however shown that this level is often difficult to determine and there is variation in assessment of vertebral levels between different operators (Broadbent 2000).
• Full aseptic technique should be observed.
• Infiltrate local anaesthetic.
• Stabilize skin over selected interspace using left hand (if right handed). See photo Figure 7.4a.
• Insert introducer needle at midpoint of L3/4 interspace and advance at slight cephalad angle through skin, subcutaneous tissue, supraspinous ligament, until stable in interspinous ligament
• Insert 25G or 27G atraumatic spinal needle through introducer needle
• Needle will pass into interspinous ligament and on to ligamentum flavum then dura.
  ○ A loss of resistance should be felt on passing through ligamentum flavum and dura.
• Withdraw stylet and watch for CSF flowing down needle and into the hub.
  ○ If blood stained allow the CSF to clear before injecting.
  ○ If it does not clear do not inject. Resite the needle.
• Stabilize hub of spinal needle to avoid movement of the needle in or out on attachment of the syringe or movement during subsequent injection.

- Attach pre–prepared syringe with dose of local anaesthetic +/– opiate.
- Inject dose.
- Withdraw needle.
- Apply dressing.
- Lie patient down if spinal inserted with patient sitting.

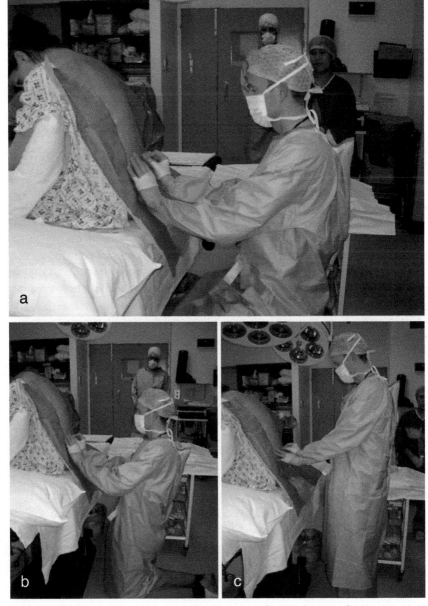

Figure 7.4 Different positions for operator on insertion of spinal (also transferable to epidural insertion).

Important points/cautions

- Always allow the cleaning solution used to dry prior to insertion of the needle through the skin.
  - There is a risk, albeit a small one, of introducing cleaning solution into the epidural or intrathecal space resulting in neurotoxicity (Scott 2009).
- Any pain, especially shooting pain into leg, suggests the needle is touching a nerve and it should therefore be withdrawn immediately.

Tips and advice

- The positioning of the operator is also important and different people will find different positions more comfortable. Try standing, sitting or kneeling and adjusting the height of the bed accordingly.
- If bone is encountered as the needle advances it is either too lateral or in the wrong vertical plane.
  - As a rule a slight cephalad approach, even in the lumbar area, is more likely to pass directly into the space.
  - If difficulty locating CSF then withdraw needle to skin and then redirect needle methodically, first aiming more cephalad then caudal.
  - If still unable withdraw needle completely and change skin insertion point by 1 cm and reattempt.
  - If still difficulty try alternative interspace or call for senior help.
- The importance of good positioning should not be underestimated. An 'easy' back can be made into a very difficult spinal with poor positioning, as can a 'difficult' back be made into an easier spinal with good positioning.
- Some anaesthetists advocate the aspiration of CSF into the syringe prior to injection of local anaesthetic +/− opiates, in order to confirm correct position.
  - Be aware that this may lead to aspiration of CSF, but may also lead to withdrawal of the spinal needle from the subarachnoid space in the process.
    - Ensure the needle doesn't move on aspiration if this technique is used.
- Be aware of the location of the hole at the end of a Whitacre needle.
  - This is proximal to the 'tip' of the needle and therefore loss of resistance can be felt without flow of CSF if inserted **very** slowly.
    - Loss of CSF flow can occur due to minimal needle migration if hole is very close to dura.
      - The hole can straddle the dura and result in poor block due to a partial spinal dose with remainder of dose going into the extradural (epidural) space.

References/further reading

Broadbent CR, Maxwell WB, Ferrie R, Wilson DJ, Gawne−Cain M, Russell R (2006). Ability of anaesthetists to identify a marked lumbar interspace. *Anaesthesia*, 55 p. 1122−6.

Scott M, Stones J and Payne N (2009). Antiseptic solutions for central neuraxial blockade: which concentration of chlorhexidine in alcohol should we use? *British Journal of Anaesthesia* 103 p. 456−7.

Epidural anaesthesia/analgesia

- Epidural analgesia is widely used for intra- and postoperative analgesia for major abdominal, vascular, thoracic and orthopaedic surgery.
- Also commonly used on labour ward where epidural analgesia for labour can be extended to provide anaesthesia for operative delivery.
- Opioids are about 10 times more potent when delivered via the epidural route compared with the intravenous route.
- A combination of opioid and local anaesthetic is typically given via the epidural route.
- Ensure adequate staffing and facilities exist on the post operative ward to ensure that patients with epidurals in situ are optimally managed.
- It is probably safer to insert epidurals in patients when they are awake.
  - Patients may complain of nerve root pain on needle or catheter insertion prompting withdrawal, or may provide advice with finding the midline of their backs!

Indications

- Intraoperative and postoperative analgesia.
  - Lumbar epidurals can provide analgesia for lower abdominal or perineal surgery.
  - Thoracic epidurals can provide analgesia for upper abdominal procedures and some thoracic procedures.
- Operative anaesthesia.
  - Rarely used alone.
- Labour analgesia.
- Epidural blood patch.
  - Following accidental, or intentional, dural puncture.
- Therapeutic injection of drugs:
  - e.g. local anaesthetic and steroids for treatment of back pain.

Contraindications

Absolute

- Patient refusal
- Severe coagulopathy
  - INR > 1.5
- Raised ICP
- Local sepsis at needle puncture site
- Thrombocytopenia
  - Different institutions and physicians have different 'cut-offs' in terms of the lowest platelet count at which they would perform an epidural. This is usually in the range of 70–100x10^9/L. **If the platelet count is less than 100x10^4/l, discuss with your consultant.**

Relative

- Systemic anticoagulation
  - Local policies vary with regards to low molecular weight heparin, heparin infusions and oral anticoagulants such as warfarin, aspirin and clopidogrel.
- Systemic sepsis
  - Increased risk of subsequent epidural abscess formation or meningitis
- Known cardiovascular disease
  - Especially aortic stenosis, mitral stenosis, pulmonary hypertension

- Previous back surgery due to anticipated technical difficulty
- Hypovolaemia
  - As risk of exaggerated hypotension
- Coagulopathy
  - Intra/extradural bleeding may occur resulting in epidural haematoma and neurological compromise
- Existing neurological deficit or disease
  - e.g. multiple sclerosis/congenital deficits
- Agitated/uncooperative patient

Complications

- Failure
- Accidental dural puncture
- Post dural puncture headache
- Neurological injury
  - Any pain radiating to legs during insertion should be taken seriously
  - Withdraw needle and reposition
- Intravascular injection
- Urinary retention
- Epidural haematoma
- Infection
  - Meningitis or epidural abscess
- Backache

Technical complications

- Failure to thread catheter
- Blood in catheter
- 'Patchy block', missed segments
- Dural puncture

Equipment

- Antiseptic solution
- Sterile procedure pack (most hospitals have specific packs available)
- 1% lidocaine and 25G needle for skin infiltration
- Epidural pack containing:
  - 16G (or 18G) epidural Tuohy needle
  - 10 ml 'loss of resistance' syringe
  - Epidural catheter
    - Controversy remains with regard to use of catheters with single vs. multiple orifices at the distal end (Dickson 1997), and as to the optimal flexibility of the catheter (Spiegel 2009).
  - Filter
- Dressing and method of securing catheter to skin
  - There are a number of methods ranging from simple tape to specific devices that attach to both the patient's skin and the catheter.
- Appropriate drugs for injection via epidural
  - Local anaesthetic +/- opiates

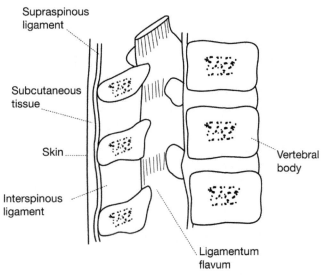

Figure 7.5 Lumbar spine anatomy for epidural insertion.

Sites/anatomical considerations

- Within the spinal canal the cord extends down to L1–2 level.
- Below this extend the fimbriae, which are relatively mobile and therefore unlikely to be damaged by the introduction of a spinal needle. Therefore the L3/4 lumbar level is most frequently chosen to insert the needle.
  - This level can be identified by determining the level of Tuffier's line, the line joining the posterior superior iliac spines, that overlies the L3/4 interspace or L4 vertebrae.
- Consider the dermatomal level of the surgical incision for the planned procedure.
  - Discuss with the surgical team if unsure.
  - The catheter should be placed at the vertebral level corresponding to the dermatomal level at the mid point of the surgical incision (see Figure 7.6).
  - T8–9 for upper abdominal procedures.
  - T10–11 for lower abdominal procedures.
  - L3–4 for labour analgesia or lower limb analgesia.

Insertion technique

- Prepare equipment and explain procedure to patient.
  - Lay out equipment in the order that it will be used.
  - Flush the catheter with saline to ensure distal lumen patency.
- Attach patient to appropriate monitoring (see section on monitoring).
- Insert intravenous cannula and attach to intravenous fluid via giving set.
- Preload with fluid if appropriate.
  - Recent NICE guidelines suggest that the practice of routine preloading with fluid in labour prior to epidural siting is unnecessary (NICE 2007).
- Position the patient as in previous section.
- Identify desired insertion point.
  - The L3/4 interspace is identified as discussed above.

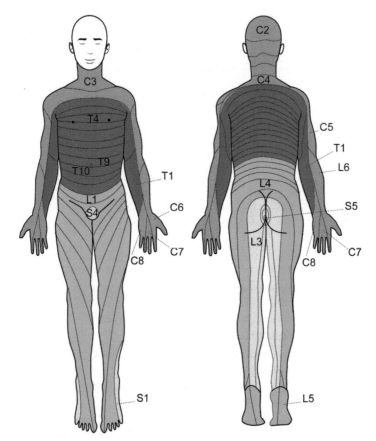

Figure 7.6 Dermatome map.

- The required thoracic interspace can be located by counting up from the L3/4 interspace or counting down from either C7 (the most prominent cervical vertebrae) or the T7 level which is at the level of the lower border of the scapula.
- Full aseptic technique.
- Infiltrate local anaesthetic.
- Stabilize skin over selected interspace using left hand, if right handed .
- Insert Tuohy needle at midpoint of chosen vertebral interspace and advance at slight cephalad angle through skin, subcutaneous tissue and supraspinous ligament, until stabilized in interspinous ligament.
- Remove the needle stylet and attach the loss of resistance syringe (filled with saline).
- Advance the needle forward maintaining pressure on the barrel of the syringe.
  - The bevel should point cephalad.
  - There are many methods used for holding the needle and syringe. (see Figure 7.8).
- There is often an increase in resistance felt as the needle tip enters the ligamentum flavum.
- On passing through the ligamentum flavum there will be loss of resistance to pressure on the syringe plunger and fluid will enter the epidural space.

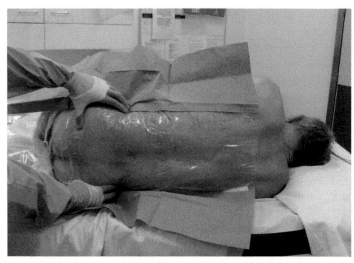

Figure 7.7 Lateral positioning for spinal or epidural insertion. Hands indicate position of the posterior superior iliac spines.

- Remove the syringe from the needle and look for free flow of either blood or clear fluid (either saline or CSF).
  - See below for options if this occurs.
- Insert epidural catheter into needle.
- Catheter should advance freely.
  - If difficult to advance consideration should be given to resiting the needle.

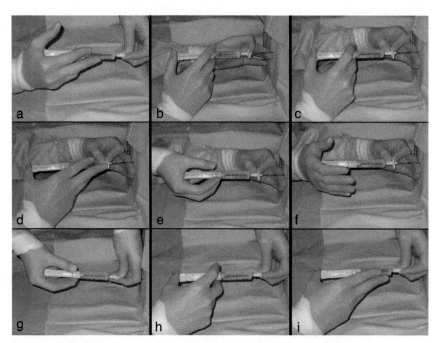

Figure 7.8 Different positions to hold hands for epidural insertion A variety of different ways which have been advocated for holding the Tuohy needle and syringe during epidural insertion. 7.7g. shows the 'Doughty' technique.

- Aim to leave between 2–5 cm (depending on personal preference) of catheter in the epidural space.
- Insert the catheter until the 12–15 cm mark appears at the proximal end of the epidural needle.
  - 2 cm of catheter in the space increases the risk of the catheter falling out.
  - With increasing lengths in the epidural space, the risk of the catheter passing out of the epidural space via an intervertebral foramen increases.
    - Results in a failed, patchy or one sided block.
- Carefully withdraw the epidural needle without dislodging the catheter.
  - Some anaesthetists advocate inserting the catheter further than desired final length in order to prevent accidental removal. Others believe that this may result in tract formation out of an intervertebral foramen resulting in a suboptimal block.
- Connect the proximal end of the catheter to the locking device and bacterial filter.
- Pull catheter back to the required distance at the skin.
  - In obese patients it is wise to then ask them to sit up.
    - The catheter is often 'pulled in' some distance and if secured before sitting up the catheter may instead be pulled out of the epidural space.
- Gently aspirate on the catheter using a 2 ml syringe to check for blood or CSF flow.
- Secure the catheter to the skin.
  - There are many methods of doing this.
    - These range from simple sterile dressings to more complicated fixation devices.
    - The method used will be dictated by local preference and protocols.

Problems on epidural insertion

- Dural puncture
  - Free flow of CSF via epidural needle indicates inadvertent dural puncture.
    - If this occurs, the choice is either to thread the catheter into the subarachnoid space and treat it as a spinal catheter, or to remove the catheter and resite at the same or another intervertebral level.
    - Caution will obviously be required in either case.
    - In labour, analgesia may not be as good as expected with a spinal catheter due to the final position of the catheter in the CSF but might reduce the incidence of dural puncture headache if left in place. The catheter promotes inflammatory changes around the site of the puncture.
    - It is unlikely that a spinal catheter would be safe for use for postoperative analgesia.
    - Resiting the catheter risks repeat dural puncture and theoretically local anaesthetic solution may be able to pass from the epidural space to the intrathecal space resulting in abnormal or extensive sensory (+/− motor) block.
  - Unrecognized dural puncture and administration of drugs intended for epidural use into the intrathecal space may result in a 'total spinal.'
    - A rapidly rising block of fast onset will be noticed, resulting in difficulty coughing and breathing, loss of upper limb strength, respiratory paralysis, cardiovascular depression and unconsciousness with fixed dilated pupils.
    - Management involves:
      - recognizing the cause, maintaining airway and ventilation (an ETT may be required) and administering cardiovascular support.

- despite loss of consciousness, some advocate the administration of addition anaesthesia in the event of tracheal intubation.
- ventilation will be required until return of adequate spontaneous ventilation and consciousness.

- Blood in needle or catheter
  - This indicates puncture of an epidural blood vessel.
  - Blood from the epidural needle should prompt removal of the needle and reinsertion.
  - Blood on aspiration of the catheter suggests that the catheter has been passed into an epidural blood vessel but may also indicate local blood vessel trauma.
    - Withdraw the catheter by 1–2 cm (if catheter length allows).
    - Flush the catheter with saline and reattempt aspiration.
    - Aspiration of frank blood again would suggest placement in a vein and it should be removed. Aspiration of blood stained saline suggests local trauma and not placement within a vein.
  - Remove a catheter if there remains **any** doubt about whether it may be sited within a blood vessel.
    - Risk of delivering a toxic intravascular dose of local anaesthetic, as well as the risk of failure of the block.

- CSF in catheter
  - Inadvertent dural puncture may not be obvious at time of insertion of the epidural needle.
    - Aspiration of clear fluid at any time must be treated as possible CSF aspiration.
  - Test the fluid for glucose using a urine or blood testing stick.
    - A positive result indicates the fluid is CSF (rather than saline) and the catheter should be removed.

- Difficulty threading catheter
  - If unable to pass beyond tip of needle (i.e. no further than 10 cm at proximal end of epidural needle, if using a 10 cm needle) then remove and flush a few millilitres of saline down the needle to try to expand the epidural space.
    - Alternatively, if not already using, reinsert using the introducer provided. This is inserted into the proximal end of the epidural needle in order to keep the catheter in a straight line at this point allowing more pressure to be exerted along the length of the catheter.
      - Be aware that this may increase the risk of placement of the catheter within the intrathecal space.
  - It may be necessary to reinsert the epidural needle in a more cephalad direction in order to reduce the angle the catheter is required to turn inside the epidural space.

- Subdural block
  - A subdural block occurs when the catheter lies between the dura mater and the arachnoid space.
  - Clinically it is sometimes difficult to identify, but characteristically the block (if inserted for labour analgesia) may:
    - be of slow onset
    - be patchy or asymmetrical
    - extend to the cervical nerves and may even result in Horner's syndrome.

○ If suspected the catheter should be resited.

■ If a subdural catheter is topped up for an operative delivery on labour ward the resulting nerve block is likely to be very unpredictable and may even result in a 'total spinal. This may be a slow insidious onset with a gradually ascending block.'

• Possibly due to the increasing volume rupturing the arachnoid mater.

Important points/cautions

• Never remove the catheter through the needle once inserted as this creates the possibility of shearing off a portion of catheter.
  ○ Remove both catheter and needle together.
• Treat every epidural dose of local anaesthetic as a 'test' dose.
  ○ Aspirate the catheter before injection to check for aspiration of blood or CSF.
• Always allow the cleaning solution on the skin to dry prior to inserting the needle.
  ○ There is a risk, albeit small, of introducing cleaning solution into the epidural or intrathecal space resulting in neurotoxicity.
• Pain, especially radiating down either or both legs, on insertion of either the needle or the catheter suggests incorrect placement affecting a nerve.
  ○ Remove and reinsert.

Tips and advice

• As previously, if bone is encountered as the needle advances it is either too lateral or in the wrong vertical plane.
  ○ As a rule, a slight cephalad approach, even in the lumbar area, is more likely to pass directly into the space.
  ○ If locating CSF is difficult then withdraw needle to skin and redirect methodically, first aiming more cephalad then more caudal.
  ○ If still no success: withdraw needle completely and change skin insertion point by 1 cm and reattempt.
  ○ If still difficulty: try alternative interspace or call for senior help.
• The importance of good positioning should not be underestimated.
  ○ An 'easy' back can become a very difficult epidural with poor positioning, as a 'difficult' back can be made into an easier epidural with good positioning.
• The paramedian approach to the epidural space is sometimes used and this can be particularly helpful if difficulty siting the epidural in the midline.
  ○ Identify the appropriate space as above and then identify the spinous process below.
  ○ Identify a point 2 cm lateral to this point as the insertion point.
  ○ Insert the needle, aiming for the midline.
  ○ As described above, use a loss of resistance technique to identify the epidural space.

References/further reading

Yentis SM, Barnes PK (2005). Snippet. Anaesthesia, 60 p. 406

Dickson MA, Moores C, McClure JH (1997). Comparison of single, end–holed and multi–orifice extradural catheters when used for continuous infusion of local anaesthetic during labour. British Journal of Anaesthesia, 79 p. 297–300

Doughty A (2005). Paternity of the Doughty technique. Anaesthesia, 60 p. 1242–3

National Institute of Clinical Excellence (2007). Intrapartum care: management and delivery of care to women in labour, guideline CG55. http://guidance.nice.org.uk/CG55

Reynolds F (2005). Hand positions and the 'son–of–Doughty' technique. *Anaesthesia*, 60 p. 717–8.

Spiegel JE, Vasudevan A, Li Y and Hess PE (2009). A randomized prospective study comparing two flexible epidural catheters for labour analgesia. *British Journal of Anaesthesia*, 103 p. 400–5.

Epidural analgesia troubleshooting

- This is intended to be a brief summary of how to approach an epidural that is not working adequately when reviewed postoperatively or on labour ward.
- This is a **brief** guide only, not an exhaustive review, which we consider to be beyond the remit of this book.

A guide for how to assess a poorly functioning epidural

- Review history of patient and documentation of insertion of the epidural.
  - Is there any opiate in the local anaesthetic?
- Ask about epidural effectiveness.
  - Has it been effective at all?
  - Any missed segments?
- Ask about current effectiveness.
  - Is there any analgesia?
  - Examine epidural pump to ensure local anaesthetic solution is being correctly administered.
- Examine the patient.
  - 'Routine' observations.
  - Urine output (urinary retention can cause breakthrough pain).
  - Examine epidural insertion site.
    - Has the catheter migrated out, assessed from the length of catheter at the skin?
    - Is local anaesthetic tracking back along catheter and leaking from insertion point?
    - Sensory block to cold? (using ice or ethyl chloride spray)
    - Check for upper level of block, missed segments and for any unilateral block.
    - Feel both feet.
      - A well functioning epidural usually results in warm, dry feet.
- Assess analgesic requirements of the patient. It might be that the epidural is no longer required and alternative forms of analgesia can be used – simple analgesics or opiate based patient controlled analgesia.
- A summary of management options can be seen in Table 7.1 below.
  - Any bolus given via the epidural catheter should be given as if it was a test dose.
  - Ensure patient is cardiovascularly stable before administering any further doses of local anaesthetic.
- Replace epidural.

Table 7.1 Management options for failed epidural block

Degree of failure of block	Description of block	Suggested action
Global failure		
Global failure	No detectable block to cold	Give up to 10 ml 0.25% bupivacaine or up to 20 ml 0.1% bupivacaine with 2 mcg/ml fentanyl.
Continued global failure despite above	No detectable block to cold	Resite epidural or use alternative analgesia.
Partial failure		
Missed segment*	Often pain felt in groin and will be one sided	If true missed segment then opiate (fentanyl 50–100 mcg) may help due to intrathecal action). Otherwise treat as for unilateral block.
Unilateral block	One sided pain. Feel feet, often one side warm and dry while painful side cold	Consider withdrawing catheter 1–2 cm if sufficient catheter in epidural space. Top up with patient in lateral position, painful side down. Give up to 10 ml 0.25% bupivacaine (consider adding 50–100 mcg fentanyl if not previously given) or up to 20 ml 0.1% bupivacaine with 2 mcg/ml fentanyl. Resite epidural if above actions fail or use alternative analgesia.
Back pain	Often associated with occipitoposterior position of the fetus in labour	Explain cause. Top up as above with local anaesthetic +/− opiate. Resiting epidural unlikely to help but if considered due to doubts over efficacy of epidural consider siting a combined spinal epidural.
Perineal pain	Associated with later stages of labour due to slower analgesia of sacral nerves in recently sited epidurals	Check sacral block and ensure bladder empty. Explain cause. Top up as above with local anaesthetic +/− opiate. Resiting epidural unlikely to help but if considered due to doubts over efficacy of epidural consider siting a combined spinal epidural.

*True 'missed segments' are uncommon and more often a unilateral block or inadequate block on one side.

Intracranial pressure monitoring

- Raised ICP can cause global cerebral ischaemia.
- Normal ICP is 5–12 mmHg.
- Management of raised ICP aims to treat the cause (if possible) and to prevent ischaemia by ensuring adequate cerebral perfusion pressure (CPP).
- In severe head injury, an average ICP > 25mmHg is associated with a twofold increase in risk of death.

  CPP = MAP – ICP (where MAP is mean arterial pressure).

  Therefore in the face of a raised ICP, the MAP can be increased to improve CPP. In addition, measures can be taken to reduce the ICP.
- In order to manage a patient with raised ICP optimally, direct measurement of ICP is essential.
- Several devices and techniques exist.
- Specific ICP waveform patterns can be identified during continuous monitoring, and these aid management (see Figure 7.9).
  - A–waves are plateau waves. Usually 50–100 mmHg, of 5–15 minutes duration. They are associated with raised ICP and compromised cerebral blood flow (CBF).
    - The frequency of occurrence of A–waves is associated with neurological deterioration and reduction in the baseline ICP reduces the frequency of the A–waves.

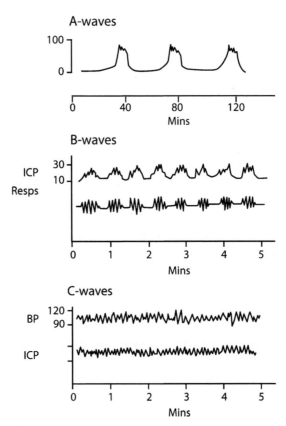

Figure 7.9 ICP waveforms.

○ B−waves are small changes in ICP. Often associated with breathing and may be due to local variations in partial pressure of O_2 and CO_2.

○ C−waves are low amplitude oscillations, around 5 per minute and are associated with variation in vasomotor tone.

○ A−waves are of value in assessing and treating raised ICP. Neither B nor C−waves are of use clinically.

Indications

- There is no list of absolute indications.
  ○ ICP monitoring is not available in all hospitals.
  ○ Staff must be familiar with the equipment and be able to interpret the results.
  ○ The following are situations when ICP monitoring should be considered.
- Any situation where therapy is targeted at manipulating ICP and CPP.
- Situations where clinical signs used to monitor ICP are obscured.
  ○ Usually by drugs
  ○ GCS < 8
- Traumatic brain injury with abnormal CT brain and reduced GCS.
- Following intracranial haemorrhage.
- Postoperative cerebral oedema.
- Acute live failure with coma.
- Metabolic conditions with raised ICP
  ○ e.g. Reye's syndrome.

Contraindications

- Uncorrected coagulopathy
- Meningitis or localized infection at insertion site
- Septicaemia

Complications

- Infection
- Intracerebral haemorrhage
  ○ Alert the neurosurgical team
- Trauma to brain parenchyma
- Blocked bolt/catheter and inaccurate calibration will lead to artificially high or low readings.

Sites and equipment

- There are four methods of measuring ICP (see Figure 7.10).
  ○ Intraventricular drain
  ○ Subarachnoid bolt or screw
  ○ Transducer−tipped systems
  ○ Epidural probe

Equipment required depends upon which method is to be used.

- ICP monitors are usually inserted by neurosurgeons, although some intensive care physicians place subarachnoid bolts.
- Strict aseptic technique should be utilized to reduce the risk of introducing infection.
- Intraventricular drain
  ○ A neurosurgical procedure.
  ○ An external pressure transducer is connected to a catheter placed in the ventricular system.

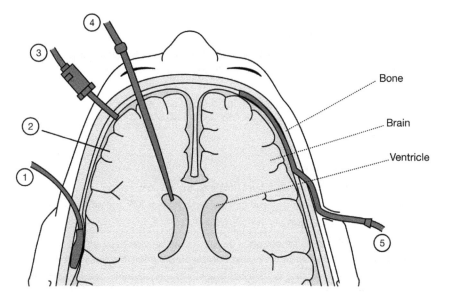

Bone

Brain

Ventricle

1. Epidural probe
2. Intraparenchymal transducer
3. Subarachnoid 'bolt'
4. Intraventricular drain
5. Subdural transducer

Figure 7.10 Sites for ICP monitoring.

- Requires an atmospheric pressure reference that should be 'zeroed' to account for movements of the patient's head position.
- Additional advantages include:
  - ability to drain CSF
  - sampling of CSF for culture.
- Risk of infection is increased after 5 days.
- Air, blood or debris in the ventricles or catheter can affect measurement.
- Subarachnoid bolt or screw
  - Usually inserted by a neurosurgeon.
  - Involves use of a fluid−coupled device, a 'bolt.'
  - Placed via a burrhole so the tip lies in the subarachnoid space.
  - Easier and quicker to place than an intraventricular drain.
  - Lower infection rates than intraventricular drains.
  - Tip can become plugged with blood or debris and this may cause inaccurate measurements.
    - This may require flushing of the system.
    - Use 0.1−0.2 ml of preservative−free saline using a 1 ml syringe.
  - The measured pressure reflects the pressure at the tip of the device and may not always be a true reflection of the ICP.
  - No ability to sample CSF.
  - Requires frequent calibration.

- Transducer tipped systems
  - A neurosurgical procedure.
  - Inserted through an airtight support bolt or via a burrhole/craniotomy.
  - Transducers are usually placed subdurally or intraparenchymally (usually in a frontal lobe).
  - Infection is a risk, but less so than with intraventricular drains.
  - The transducer measures localized ICP around the tip, and this may not always represent global ICP.
- Epidural probe
  - The least invasive system.
  - Fibreoptic sensor placed via a burr hole into the epidural space.
  - Uncertainty exists about the true correlation between ICP and epidural pressure.

Important points/cautions

- Any problems with an ICP monitoring device should be discussed with a neurosurgeon and the critical care physician responsible for the patient's care.
- When manipulating, flushing or redressing any of the equipment aseptic technique must be employed to reduce the risk of introducing infection.
- When intraventricular drains are connected to an external drainage system, care must be taken to ensure the 'zero level' of the system remains at the reference point (usually the external auditory meatus) as CSF drainage will either increase or decrease if the level is altered.
- A transducer system is connected to the bolt or the ventricular drain and it is possible to have a three way tap in the system to allow continuous pressure monitoring and intermittent CSF drainage or vice versa. **No intraflow device should be used.**

Index

References to page numbers in **bold typeface** indicate a figure or table.